3 Steps To YOUR BEST BODY in record time

Published by CelebrityPress™, Orlando, FL
A division of The Celebrity Branding Agency®

Celebrity Branding® is a registered trademark
Printed in the United States of America.

ISBN: 978-0-9833404-0-9
LCCN: 2011922320

For more information, please write:

CelebrityPress™,
520 N. Orlando Ave, #2,
Winter Park, FL 32789

or call 1.877.261.4930

Visit us online at www.**CelebrityPressPublishing**.com

3 Steps To YOUR BEST BODY in record time

America's Leading Fitness Experts Reveal The

Proven 3-Step System

To The Body You Always Wanted

...In Minimum Time

TABLE OF CONTENTS

STEP 3 – FITNESS

FOREWORD

I've been fortunate to be a co-author of 2 best-selling books on health, fitness, and personal development in my lifetime. But neither of those publications compare to the release of this book and what it has to offer the world.

Over the last 10 years, my business (and life) has transformed from that of a fitness coach to studio owner, then to multi-location studio owner, and now to the owner of company called NPE – that supports entrepreneurs in growing their businesses in the fitness industry.

And today I have the pleasure of working with thousands of fitness and nutrition coaches from around the world in growing their businesses. This book is the latest chapter (pun intended) in supporting the "cream of the crop" fitness professionals in getting the word out about what they do.

The authors who've contributed to this book are NOT "reality TV" coaches. They are the real deal. Each of them has invested thousands of hours in working with clients of all backgrounds and levels, to accomplish their personal health and fitness goals.

What you will read in these pages is NOT theory. **These are proven methods for getting the results you want.**

I encourage you to pay close attention to the words on each page, but don't let yourself get stuck there. If you're serious about accomplishing a health and fitness goal or making a change in your life, then TAKE ACTION NOW!

Pick up the phone and give one of these experts a call. Visit their web-sites. Stop by their facilities.

Your best body awaits you just around the corner!

To your success,

Sean Greeley
President
NPE, LLC

STEP 1

MINDSET

CHAPTER 1

FIVE STEPS TO ACHIEVING ANY HEALTH AND FITNESS GOAL

BY SEAN GREELEY

"Happiness lies, first of all, in health."
~ George William Curtis

To me, fitness is a way of life. Making (and keeping) a commitment to taking care of your health is critical to not only looking and feeling good, but giving your mind and body the strength it needs to reach your goals and be there for others who depend on you.

I enjoy pushing myself to work hard. My idea of relaxation is doing a Crossfit style workout until I'm nauseous. It doesn't sound like fun to many people, but, to me, achieving optimum fitness helps me to work and play at the highest level possible – and enjoy life to the fullest.

Fitness has also helped me to achieve many dreams - from being a top 400m runner in the New England Championships to being part of the USA Wakeboard team for three years and competing in both European and World Championships. I was also blessed to be able to successfully battle Stage IV cancer in 2003 and regain my complete health, to the point where I was recognized as one of the top personal trainers in the country by the American Council of Exercise in 2005.

At the same time, I've always admired systems. The right systems create success in whatever endeavor you might undertake – and it's helped me build a multi-million dollar business from the ground up. If there's a faster, easier and more profitable way to do something, I'll usually find it.

Since two of my big passions are systems and fitness, it was a natural next step to put them together to help people reap the benefits of good health as I have throughout my life. You may be one of the millions who are sick and tired of being… well, sick and tired. If so, this chapter will introduce you to my 5-step system – and give you the structure to begin turning around your health.

Let me share with you the 5 steps you can take to reach any fitness goal you have and live a better quality of life. These are the same 5 steps I've personally coached thousands of clients through when they make the commitment to feeling and looking better. Although I only have time to give you the broad strokes here, they will provide you with the basic blueprint to achieve your goals.

STEP ONE: DEFINE YOUR GOALS, MOTIVATION AND COMMITMENT

Your mindset is all-important whenever you face any challenge – and improving your fitness is certainly no different. If anything, it's *more* important to be clear in your mind about what you want to achieve.

Start with your **goals**. If you're like most of the fitness clients I've worked with over the years, you're looking to reduce body fat, drop some weight, improve muscle tone and definition, increase your strength, and just develop a healthier lifestyle overall that leads to more energy and better vitality. But spend a few minutes getting more specific about those goals. Ask yourself these questions:

- If you want to lose weight, how much weight do you want to lose?

- If you want to build more muscle, how much muscle do you want to gain?
- If you want to improve your strength, by how much do you want to improve?

If you only have a more general goal, such as to just be healthier and feel better, that's fine – but a few specifics would help. This is the point when you should write down those specific goals – it may sound silly, but research shows that writing down goals, instead of just thinking or saying them, gives you more inner strength to achieve them.

Once you've written down those goals, think about WHY those goals are important to you. You must have a strong **motivation** to achieve them – understanding that motivation is key to moving forward.

For many folks that are new to fitness, they just want to improve their quality of life. Their weight has gradually gone up over the past few years, and the little things they've tried in the past to lose weight (like no longer drinking alcohol or cutting out the junk food) just aren't working anymore. They know it's time to do this thing right.

Other people are already in a program that just isn't giving them the results they want. Or they might have a special event coming up, like a wedding, a reunion, or a birthday party of note where they want to look their best.

Whatever your reason why, it has to be strong. So take time for some personal reflection and understand why you're doing this.

If you have your goals and your motivation worked out, you should now move on to your commitment. How committed are you to achieving your goals? Give yourself a personal ranking on a commitment scale from 1 to 10, with a "10" meaning you're willing to do "whatever it takes" to accomplish your goals.

Here's a little secret – if you view your commitment as anything less than that "10," you're not going to be very successful. So, whatever number you assigned to your commitment, ask yourself why you chose it.

Many people give themselves lower scores because they struggle with knowing what to do to be successful. Maybe they don't know how to implement proper nutrition or manage their time so that they keep their exercise appointments. This is where a coach or trainer can really be of use – they hold you accountable, give you the knowledge you need to make a program work, and provide the support to lead you through to success.

STEP TWO: PERFORM AN INITIAL EVALUATION

This is where you find your starting point. It's important to know where you began so you can measure your progress along the way. You can have a trainer help you with this, or perform a simple Fitness Assessment on your own. Either way the assessment should include measuring the things you seek to change. For example:

- Weighing yourself on a scale
- Taking some measurements of your body
- Taking a body fat assessment (which many scales now offer today as a built-in calculation)
- Completing a profile of your current nutrition habits
- Taking some "before" photographs of your body

Now, let me say that I don't know *anyone* who enjoys doing an assessment of their body, particularly when they're already unhappy about where they are. But try to get past that and do it anyway.

The photos may be the hardest part. While nobody likes to look at a less-than-desirable photograph of themselves, some initial "before" photos will provide you with a great reference in the future for those times when you say, "I don't feel like anything's happening." Comparing a photograph of yourself every three to six weeks will allow you to *really start seeing changes occur* and *you'll get excited about the results*. That way you'll be more motivated to continue with your program and do everything-it-takes to be successful in achieving your goals.

STEP THREE: DESIGN YOUR PROGRAM

Steps 1 and 2 helped you decide where you want to go and locked down where you're starting from. Now it's time to connect the dots and plot your course. You need to create a road map to get you from where you are now to where you want to be.

This may be a little difficult to do on your own, as it requires a wide knowledge of fitness and nutrition. Let me share with you what I call the "The Six Proven Components of Success."

1. **Nutrition-** the foundation of all health and fitness
2. **Supplementation-** to fill in the voids in your nutrition program
3. **Resistance training**- to build lean muscle and ramp up the metabolism
4. **Cardiovascular exercise-** to optimize fat burning and heart health
5. **Flexibility**- to prevent injury and promote recovery from exercise
6. **Coaching-** knowledge, support and accountability to get you to the finish line

1. We'll start with #1 – **nutrition.** Nutrition is the foundation of all health and fitness. I work with my clients to create meal plans and make a grocery list of the foods that are helpful. You should have an *exact plan of what you need to eat* in a day to be successful – and then simply check off those items as you go through your day. If the plan is solid and you follow it, you're going to see results.

2. Once you start eating better, you'll find that your energy will increase and your metabolism will start working again. You also, however, need to address the second component, **supplementation,** to fill in the voids in your diet and provide your body with the nutrients you're not getting from your food.

   There are three main supplements I recommend to all of my clients. Number one is a good multi-vitamin/mineral supplement. Why? Because every major medical and health organization in America today now recommends you take a multi-vitamin/ multi-mineral supplement for complete nutrition. In addition to a good multi-vitamin/mineral supplement, we also recommend additional anti-oxidants like vitamin C, vitamin E, an additional B-complex and, unless you're eating a ton of red meat, additional iron.

   I also recommend using a meal replacement product to all of my clients because I don't know anyone who can realistically eat a complete meal six times a day and have a normal life. That's why having the convenience of a good, balanced meal-replacement shake or bar is great in between your major meals, or even for breakfast-on-the-go.

Third, I recommend having a post-workout recovery shake. After your resistance training or strength training workout, a recovery shake is critical to transferring your muscles into the recovery phase. Putting your body into the recovery phase fast allows you to reduce muscle soreness and start rebuilding and repairing tissue right away. That way you can maximize the effort you put in at the gym and get the best results from your workout in the shortest period of time.

3. Let's look at our third "Component of Success" – **resistance training**, the first part of our exercise regimen. Your resistance training program should be designed to build lean muscle, get your metabolism going, and increase your strength. I recommend a combination of functional-type and weight-type training exercises. That way, you're challenging your body completely - not just the big muscles, but also the little ones, so they can actually support your body, the way you move in the real world.

4. Now, let's move on to **cardiovascular exercise.** You want to focus on this for heart health and to optimize your body's ability to burn fat 24/7. As a general rule, for good health and weight management, everyone should aim for at least three non-consecutive days of cardiovascular activity each week. Traditional cardio includes running outdoors or on a treadmill, elliptical machines, rowers, regular or stationary bikes, aerobic classes, stairsteppers, etc. Swimming, rollerblading outside, mountain biking, and cycling are all great outdoor cardio activities. But for efficiency and time effectiveness, I would encourage you to focus on INTERVAL training for your cardiovascular exercise. You can also mix up your resistance training to include intervals for a power-packed punch of intensity and efficiency.

5. Our next component is **flexibility.** You need to prepare your body for a workout every day to prevent injury, promote the recovery process and just get your body moving better again – and you need to cool down afterwards.

A good warm-up should last anywhere from 5 to 10 minutes and should include some low-intensity cardiovascular exercise, like walking on the treadmill, jogging, biking or some cardio-calisthenics. This will prepare you to then spend another 5-10 minutes performing the warm-up stretching exercises, get in tune with your body that day, and get ready to have a great workout.

Likewise, after you've done the workout, it's a MUST that you spend time cooling down. Doing so allows you to flush out lactic acid, toxins, and other waste products that are left over in your muscles from exercise. Flushing these toxins out with some light cardiovascular exercise and stretching again will reduce delayed onset muscle soreness (that feeling like you can't walk for several days), and (along with post-workout nutrition) will accelerate your body's recovery process. The cool down should also be around 5 to 10 minutes or so.

6. The final component is **coaching.** My job as a coach is to provide my clients with the knowledge to create a good program and eliminate the "guesswork" for you. My expertise comes from years of study and working hands-on in the trenches coaching my clients. I already know what works and what doesn't. You need a coach with the same level of experience who can support you through your program.

STEP FOUR: PUTTING YOUR PROGRAM INTO ACTION

Once we review our clients' plans, we make it their next step to start taking the action they need to take, in order to get the results they want. It's time to get off the bench and get in the game – and that means you have to learn the components of the program, and you have to learn new habits.

Here's a newsflash: You already have fitness and nutrition habits in your lifestyle right now; they're just habits that aren't getting you to where you want to get. It's time to change those habits out for better ones.

The first 3 weeks of program implementation are critical. Studies show that it takes around 21 days to integrate a new habit into your life. Think about it—you don't have to consciously tell yourself to brush your teeth in the morning, take a shower or get that cup of coffee when you wake up — it's just part of your routine every day.

Similarly, you want to build good habits around exercise and nutrition so you can maintain your results and always be where you want to be. If you follow this plan for 21 days, you're going to have to think about it at first to get things going. But, once you get on track, it becomes automatic. You'll be on auto-pilot with your new habits and your success will be guaranteed.

STEP FIVE: REGULARLY ASSESS YOUR RESULTS & UPDATE YOUR PROGRAM

As you progress through your program, regularly evaluate your progress and results. Doing so will allow you to gauge where you are on your "road-map", make any course corrections that are necessary, and continue to your destination. I recommend you mark on your calendar the dates (about every 3 weeks) for you to update your evaluation. Measure everything just like you did the first day of your program.

It's been proven time and time again that people always perform better, whether it's in their job or in sports, when their results are measured. That's why runners are timed, why accountants prepare monthly P/L statements, and why we keep score in football. Measuring your activity and results is an absolute must. You MUST evaluate yourself at regular intervals throughout this program. That way you can hold yourself accountable for your results, prevent any backsliding, and stay on track with your plan to achieve your goals.

Again, this chapter featured the broad strokes of the system I've shared over the years with all our clients – many of the subjects we covered here could (and should) have their own chapter. In fact, these are the exact same steps I use with other business owners today to help them grow their fitness business. The steps work to improve anything you desire… not just your health and fitness. If you visit my website at: www.FitnessMarketingMuscle.com, you'll see many testimonials as well as real "before" and "after" pictures of my clients (today they are testimonials related to business success instead of fitness results)

They're serious proof that I've gotten tremendous success stories from this program in working with my clients.

Everyone deserves a long life filled with health and happiness. Taking the right approach to fitness and nutrition helps you achieve that goal. I wish you luck in achieving all your goals and living your life to the fullest.

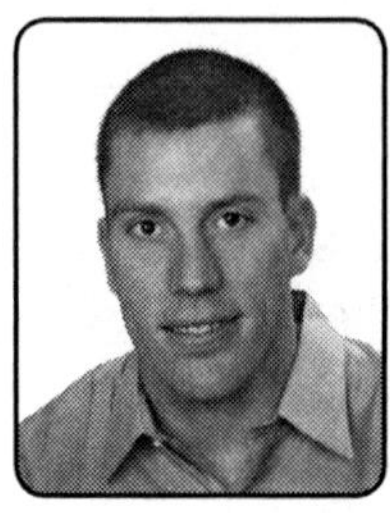

ABOUT SEAN

Sean is all about making the most from all you've got. As a professional Wake Boarder he rose to the very highest level, representing team USA at the World Championships in Germany. As a Fitness business owner, again, he far surpassed what many of his peers in the industry dreamed of accomplishing, creating a 653-strong client base in just 3 years, starting from nothing. Sean was also recognized as one of the Top 10 personal trainers in the country.

Now with NPE, Sean (along with Eric) has started a business from scratch and turned it into a multi-million dollar, industry-leading company in just two years. This feat was recognized by the very best business builders in the world at the Glazer Kennedy Info-Summit 2008 where Sean & Eric won the "Info Marketers of the Year" award.

Sean's biggest asset is his ability to systemize and then maximize almost every business essential – from sales, to marketing, to management and more. If there's a faster, easier and more profitable way to do something, Sean will find it.

In his spare time Sean likes to "relax" by cranking out nausea-inducing Cross-Fit workouts, surfing in oftentimes shark- infested waters, or being pulled at up to 23mph, hanging onto the back of a wakeboarding boat.

CHAPTER 2

MAKING ROOM FOR SELF WORTH, FITNESS AND HEALTH AT PINK IRON

BY HOLLY HOLTON & MEG ROBLES

HOLLY'S STORY:

My love for fitness began at the age of 15 in a small town in Louisiana when I picked up my first women's health and fitness magazine. I was hooked. I loved how strong the women's bodies looked, their shapely arms and six pack abs. I knew instantly that was how I wanted to look, what I wanted to be... a figure competitor. That began my daily trips to my local gym. I got a lot of advice from other "gym rats" and devoured every bit of information I could get my hands on. For years, I was the most dedicated high school-aged kid at the gym and usually the only girl in the weight room. I was smart enough to know that those fitness models in my favorite magazines got their bodies from time spent in the weight room, but I still didn't have a grasp on healthy eating. I was in shape, but I still wasn't in the "fitness model" shape that I desired, and that was because I wasn't eating properly.

2004 was a big year for me. I had a small wedding and married my college boyfriend at the age of 19. That was also the year that I finally decided to nail down my goal and become an official figure competitor. Since I never do things halfway, I decided to enter the biggest fitness show of the year, the "Miss Bikini Universe" and "Miss Fitness Model Universe." Upon deciding to do this, I realized I had eight weeks to get ready for this show – so I enlisted the help of a local bodybuilder. He helped me with the proper nutrition and a workout plan to reach my goal of getting on stage. I had never eaten like that in my life, and it quickly made me realize that my diet of Subway sandwiches and diet Coke was no longer 'going to cut it.' I reached my goal and made it to the show. I also exceeded my goal, far beyond my expectations, when I placed in the top five for both the Miss Bikini Universe and Miss Fitness Model Universe competitions. I stood right there on stage alongside many of the women I had read about in my fitness magazines since I was 15. It was exhilarating.

A few weeks later, the pictures of me on stage looked quite different to the girl who looked back at me in the mirror. What I had failed to realize was that after the show, I needed to get right back on my 'clean-eating' plan and workout routine. Thus began my years of yo-yo dieting. I would diet down to do a show, go, place well, come home, eat till my heart was content, gain weight, then do it all over again. I would pick up more and more information but never seemed able to get it quite right. During this time, my marriage was also falling apart. During the first year of marriage, my husband had been drafted into the NFL and for the following 2 years, our life was chaotic, moving around the country from team to team. This gypsy lifestyle was hard on us both. He succumbed to the pressures and temptations that go along with the NFL and our marriage was quickly over. At first I was devastated, then I was numb. In an instant, my happy little life fell apart. Wanting a fresh start, I moved to Dallas, Texas.

I knew that my true passion in life was fitness. I wanted to turn this into a career for myself so I got my personal training certification. I loved training clients and helping people. I wanted to continue doing this on a larger scale, so I packed up everything I could in my car, and on a hope and a prayer, moved to Los Angeles, California. I was 23 years old, divorced, and in a city where I knew no one. The only constant in my life, the only thing I could control at this point was my nutrition and my workouts, but I took it to the extreme. For months, I restricted calories and would do cardio for hours on end. I started to look and feel unhealthy. I lost my vision for who I wanted to be and fitness wasn't fun anymore. I was exhausted, so I took it to the opposite extreme and completely stopped everything. I immediately began to gain weight. I hated the way I felt and looked. The higher my jeans size went up, the lower my self confidence went down.

At this point, I decided that I wouldn't let life circumstances destroy my hopes and dreams. I studied, learning as much as I could about the human body and it's response to food and training. I finally understood that for years when I thought I was living "healthy", I was really hurting my body. My outlook changed and I started looking at food as fuel, not something that I should be afraid of. Once again, I saw strength-training workouts as something that was fun to do, not a chore. As I did this, I became me again, ...I regained my confidence. I learned how the body worked and how to stop the vicious cycle of 'yo-yo' dieting. My previous behavior had wreaked havoc on my metabolism, so through "clean" eating, my body began to work properly again. During this transformation and through my years as a trainer, I met so many women who faced similar issues, who had been through hard times and lost themselves in the process. They were women who looked in the mirror one day and didn't recognize the person staring back at them, ...Women who had lost their confidence. Though they were ready to make a change, these same women were also too intimidated and too embarrassed to set foot in a gym, so they entered a vicious cycle.

On a hike one day with my friend Rick, I was complaining to him about this issue. I wanted a comfortable environment for women who faced these issues to go to get the help they needed — a place where women could feel strong and empowered with no intimidation. Fitness had changed my life, ...helped to shape me into the person I am, ... saved me and gave me direction when I had none. I know not everyone's calling is fitness, heck, a lot of people hate working out, but it's the after effects that count. I believe there is nothing better than looking and feeling your best and knowing that you worked hard to feel that way. There's nothing better than the feeling of accomplishment that fitness can give you. I wanted the opportunity to spread that knowledge to others, and to help other women who have struggled with their goals to finally reach them. Rick loved the idea and helped me to build upon it; it eventually evolved into our women's only gym, Pink Iron.

MEG'S STORY:

I am one of the owners of Pink Iron, but I also consider myself a client of Pink Iron. I have a background in marketing and have never worked in a gym before. At Pink Iron, I do a lot of the financial aspects of the business, but I am also at the gym most of the day. By meeting all the trainers and ladies that come to Pink Iron, I have really been able to involve myself in the fitness world and learn a lot. I have even started to work with some of the trainers, which is great, because then I can see Pink Iron from the perspective of a client as well. I have learned so much about healthy eating and have made it a lifestyle change. I actually had never really been consistent in my workout routine and I would eat junk food like pizza and cake all the time. I would work out for a few months and then take a few months off, I just could not get into a regular routine. I looked on working out as a chore and would wait until after work to workout. I am not a morning person, so the idea of exercising before work was not appealing. After work, something more important always seemed to come up, so it was easy to skip a workout. Before I knew it, it had been months and I had not worked out. This was my pattern for years and years. Once we opened up Pink Iron, I met many women who loved to work out. They did it because it made them feel good, and feel good about themselves. I started to understand the joy of working out and pushing myself to do things that I didn't think I could do. I now enjoyed working out and I looked forward to it, but it was still difficult for me to find the time to workout on a consistent basis.

At one point, my personal life started to get very chaotic and it spiraled out of control in just about all areas. I started to feel helpless and it was hard for me to concentrate on anything. I noticed that I was becoming angry and numb to a lot of things. I wasn't my happy, carefree self anymore. I needed to change something, and I needed to change it fast.

I decided that it was finally time for me to start working out on a consistent basis. At first, my main reason was to get out some of the aggression and stress that was building up. Soon my aggression was out and I was just working out because I enjoyed it and it made me feel good. I really started to focus on my workout routine and eating well. I played around with a few different workout patterns and finally found that waking up in the morning to workout before work was the best option for me. This way I always make time for myself. I treat myself to an hour or two everyday just to focus on myself and not worry about anyone else. I am able to de-stress and get ready for my day. My mind goes blank and I just concentrate on my task at hand; it is one of the best parts of my day, and devoted solely to me. I also started working out with a buddy, so it is easier to wake up in the morning – knowing that someone is waiting for me.

Working out and eating clean started out as one of the only things I felt like I could control in my life at that time. Focusing on bettering myself really helped me to put my life in order and see that I could control many other areas of my life too. I stopped feeling helpless and started to build back my confidence. I started to really look at myself and my life, and change the things that I did not like. I started to build my life into what I wanted it to be, not the way I was accepting it to be. I am now able to focus and put myself first. Life is constantly changing and we have to change with it; keeping your confidence up makes life easier, and helps things fall into place.

HOW TO GET YOUR CONFIDENCE BACK:

Hi, Holly here again! Meg and I are so lucky to be doing what we love every day, to put our vision into action. I personally meet with every new Pink Iron client when they first start. I sit down with them to do a fitness and nutrition consultation. The first question I always ask is "What are your goals?" I get an array of answers such as: "I want to lose 10, 20, 30 pounds." "I want to tone up." "I want to be stronger." My next question is always, "Why is your goal important to you?" This question is just as important as the first. Yes, goal setting is imperative. Without a goal, there is no direction. But without knowing why you have this goal, there is no motivation to reach it. Almost without fail, the answer I get from each client for "why is your goal important to you?" is "I want to get my self-confidence back." There are many variations of it. "I want to look better." "I want to feel better about myself." "I want to be *me* again." But the answers all boil down to the same thing, regaining confidence. I hear many stories, unique to each person, about what has led them to where they are, sitting in front of me, hoping for anything that will help them. Some have tried all the fads and failed each time, they are frustrated and think that they are beyond help. Some have just reached their tipping point, the point where they are ready to finally put themselves first. Some are here for health reasons and are embarrassed that they have let it get this far. With every story that I hear, I am happy that I have been through trying times myself so I can say "I understand" and truly mean it. I then get them started on the journey to getting their self-confidence back.

SIX STEPS TO GAINING CONFIDENCE AND RAISING YOUR SELF WORTH:

1. Set your goal: We make each client set a goal. If you don't have one, find one. We like to have a date attached to each goal. The brain needs something to work towards so we establish that goal, write it down, and remind each client of their goal often.

2. Take the first step: For many people, the first step is the hardest step in a fitness program. They are intimidated or scared of failure. Once you get started, you may find that it isn't so bad after all. The feeling of accomplishment after each workout will help to boost your confidence and keep you coming back.

3. Eat: So many women believe that restricting calories is the answer. Many women eat only one meal a day and wonder why they don't lose weight. Well, here is a little secret… you actually have to eat to lose weight. When you restrict calories, your metabolism slows down, making it difficult to shed body fat. If you feed yourself small "clean" meals throughout the day (around every 3 hours), then your body will work more efficiently and help you to lose weight.

4. Eat Clean: Fuel your body with the right foods. We teach our clients to follow a clean diet of unprocessed foods. A diet that is a balance of lean proteins, complex carbohydrates,

and plenty of vegetables and fruits. When you are taking care of your body this way, it shows quickly. You will get leaner and toned. Your hair, skin, and nails will look great. You will have much more energy. All of these things will be major confidence boosters.

5. Put yourself first: Working with all women, we have many moms and wives. These are women who have gotten used to being last. When they come to us, they are tired and many times feel guilty for taking time out to do something for themselves. That's when we have to explain, if you don't take care of yourself properly, you will not be able to take care of anyone properly. What does the flight attendant on airline flights always say? *"Put on your oxygen mask first before helping others."* Set a goal to take out an hour a day a few times a week to focus on yourself and your health. The rest of your life will improve instantly.

6. Work Hard: Anything worth having is worth working hard for. We teach our clients that results aren't going to come overnight. It will take hard work and sweat to reach your goals. One thing that does come quickly is the sense of accomplishment after every hard workout. If you know you have put your all into each workout, it is an instant confidence booster.

The main thing is to just get started. Even if you're not doing a lot in the beginning, work up to doing more as time goes on, and you will be well on your way. Make up your mind that you are finally going to take care of YOU and then set your goals around that. At Pink Iron, we are constantly seeing women transform. They walk in at the beginning, unsure of themselves with their head hanging low. Within a few weeks, the same woman is confidently coming through the door with her shoulders back and a new spring in her step. She's telling her trainer, "put more weight on that barbell!" That's what keeps us inspired and motivated. **Fitness has changed our lives... now it's your turn!**

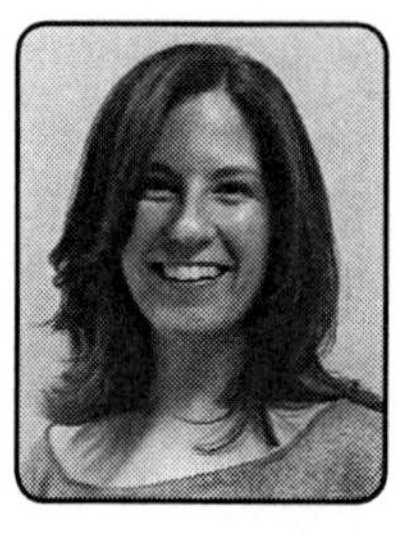

ABOUT MEG

Meg Robles is co-owner and COO of Pink Iron. She has dedicated herself to helping all Pink Iron clients reach their goals. She knows each client by name and always greets them with a friendly face. She is vital in creating Pink Iron's family atmosphere where everyone feels welcome and comfortable. There is nothing that makes her happier then when Pink Iron clients reach their goals and succeed.

Meg has always dreamed of owning her own business and was thrilled to get involved with Pink Iron from its very first day. She was instrumental in the start-up of the company and in helping it to become the flourishing business that it is today. On a day-to-day basis she works hard to drive the business forward, focusing on the business financials and first class customer service.

Meg was born and raised in Vienna, Virginia, a suburb of Washington, DC. She started swimming in her neighborhood summer swim league at age 7 and continued until age 18. During high school, she played on the women's softball and basketball teams, as well as the swim team. She also coached a girls' Little League softball team for three years. Meg has a Bachelor's of Business Administration from James Madison University in Harrisonburg, Virginia. She majored in Business Marketing and minored in Human Resources. After completing college, Meg worked in various sales and marketing positions in Northern Virginia. She was an international account manager at a direct mail firm and an investor relations coordinator at a commercial real estate firm. Meg moved to Los Angeles in 2007 and continued to work in marketing until starting Pink Iron.

Meg is an avid animal lover and is a proud Mom to her rescued cat, Desti. In her spare time, she likes to work out, watch movies, and cook.

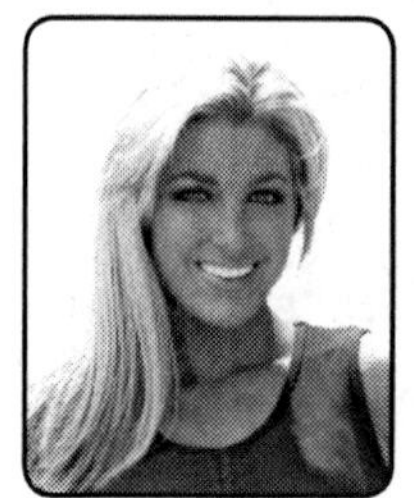

ABOUT HOLLY

Holly Holton is a Certified Personal Trainer and the owner of the women's only Pink Iron Training Studio in West Hollywood, CA, where the mission is improving women's lives through fitness.

Holly has appeared on E! Entertainment Television, Entertainment Tonight, and ABC, Fox, and NBC affiliates as a fitness expert. She has been featured in LA Confidential, LA Health News, In Touch, Genlux, and Agenda Magazines. She has also been featured on the cover of Natural Muscle magazine. She has appeared as the official trainer and spokesperson for Got Milk?'s "Get Fit with Got Milk?" program.

Growing up in Lake Charles, Louisiana, Holton's love for fitness was found by flipping through health and fitness magazines. It was at the early age of fifteen that she became aware of this passion and started going in that direction. By nineteen she had already gained world-wide recognition by placing in the top 5 athletes at the Ms. Bikini Universe and Model Universe amongst over 150 seasoned competitors. Continually competing and accomplishing personal and professional goals, Holton became known as a top contender in both the Fitness America Pageant and the World Natural Sports Organization.

It was through training fellow competitors that Holton decided to dedicate her life to improving the lives of others. It was this perseverance that fueled her move to Dallas, Texas to attend the Cooper Aerobic Institute to further her career. During this time, Holton worked as a Personal Trainer at a national chain fitness center, where she experienced how a large corporation runs and the negative effects that their clients and staff endure. It was the knowledge gained through these previous experiences that ultimately shaped her future.

With Los Angeles as the perfect backdrop to assist in achieving her ambitions, Holton relocated again to the fitness capital of America. Personal experience and public demand soon brought together Holton and her best friend Rick Robles to create what now has evolved into Pink Iron. Now living her dream of owning her own studio and spreading her love of fitness, Holton brings success and happiness to her clients by teaching strength, confidence and passion for a healthy and fit lifestyle.

CHAPTER 3

FROM 'AVERAGE JOE' TO G.I. JOE

BY GIAMPIERO "JP" MONTANARI

It's a hot summer day in 1998 back in my high school years. Today is the first day of a life-changing experience that will never let me be the same, I'm told. I put my bag down as sirens and screams calling me to formation give beginning to my seven-day journey. I'm scared and don't really know anyone in my barrack; one thought goes through my head… "Now I know why they call it 'Hell Week' here in Military Summer Camp."

I was just a 150 pound kid who wanted to do something different He wanted to prove he could be strong, and was quickly realizing it was going to take more than just a desire to be better.

My sergeant comes busting through the doors screaming, rushing and commanding us to go outside and go to the 'platoon'. "I better go outside," I said to myself, and quickly followed another kid who seemed to know what they were doing and what a 'platoon' was.

By now its about ten in the morning, my stomach is growling and I keep on asking myself, "How am I supposed to survive this week?" I'm not used to this, and to be honest, to me summer meant waking up at noon and having Frosted Flakes while watching TV in my pajamas. Well, I guess this is not going to be a regular summer, I've only been here for less than 15 minutes and I'm pretty much ready to go back to Florida and regretting signing up for it.

While having this internal fight and regrets about being there, we are all called to 'attention'. This means you stand up straight with your arms by your side, chin up, chest out and heels together making a 'V' with your feet. Nobody talks now, you could hear a pin drop, there is only one man allowed to do anything and that is the battalion commander. He is just a kid, maybe a few years older than I am, not a real military officer. But for the next few days he will be treated as one. We will honor him, follow him, obey him and above all, learn how to be a great leader.

My perception was all wrong, I thought I was there to play soldier, but I was there to be transformed, to be shaped, to be taught, to go from being an 'average Joe' to becoming a GI Joe. For many people, a soldier is someone who is part of a group of people physically trained to defend a nation and serve a country. Even though this is true, there is a lot more to it than that.

You see, that summer changed my perception not only about military training, but also about myself. I was encouraged to push my limits by changing core beliefs about myself. In those seven days, I believe I went from thinking like an 'average Joe' to behaving like GI Joe.

I come from a military background. My dad was a Navy Officer and all of my uncles on my mother's side were Army Officers as well, so being exposed to men in uniform and military bases was not strange to me. But that did not help at all. If I wanted to survive the program, I was going to have to go through it myself, and no one else could help.

How can this relate to fitness? How can a Military Summer Camp experience relate to reaching all of your fitness goals?

The fact is that it serves as a perfect example of what we experience everyday as 'average Joes'. As I mentioned before, I arrived at that camp thinking like a typical 16 year old, and I now believe that in those seven days I learned many of the leadership skills I now possess. The only way for that to happen was to make an 'inside out' change, …to stop thinking like a spoiled young 16 year old, …to stop wishing not to be there;

but the fact was that I was there, and that the ONLY option I had was to change my mindset and become the person it takes to go through it.

Fitness goals are the same. Our biggest battle is not against a food choice or fast food restaurant, our only fight should be against that 'average Joe' that we all have inside, the one that pushes us to be mediocre, lazy, and behave like society tells us we should. The fact is that this type of behavior is killing us …as individuals, …as a society, … as a nation and …as a race. If you want life-lasting change to occur, whether in your body, social habits, health or the way you feel, then an inner change must occur first – there is just no other way – and I call this the *GI Joe Mindset.*

Let's identify what I believe are the most common inner enemies we have and what I will be referring to as *Average Joe Brain.* For you to understand this analogy, you must first know that the person who you talk to and listen to the most is the biggest influence over your decisions and actions. Now, you might think this person is your wife, husband, boss, coach, pastor, etc., but the truth is that the person who you talk to and listen to the most – is *yourself.* We spend hours a day having inner conversations and many of these inner conversations come from an *Average Joe Brain*:

As a fitness professional, and in my 10 years working with people just like you, I have identified five common opinions that your Average Joe Brain believes, but are not true. You don't have to continue walking around believing these lies, but instead, replace them with the *GI Joe Mindset.*

BELIEF #1

Average Joe Brain: *"It's not my fault,"* you keep on telling yourself. A lady once told me, "I gained weight because I cook for my husband at night and I eat that food." I never heard a worst excuse. Another one told me, "I had Macaroni and Cheese for lunch because that's what my kids wanted to eat." Excuses, excuses, excuses! ***Lack of personal responsibility is one of the major reasons why things may go wrong in life, business, health, family.*** You start blaming others for your poor choices and that leads you down a never-ending road to failure.

GI Joe Mindset: Even though there are things in life that are out of our control, they don't happen every day. And when they do, it is within our control as to how we react and what we do about it. Taking responsibility for the past and present is the only road to future success. *Stop blaming others and take the right actions consistently – until you reach your desired goal.*

BELIEF #2

Average Joe Brain: *"Everyone is doing it!"* Some people never grow out of a teenager's mindset and vocabulary. Many clients use this as an excuse, trying to cover up the fact that they ate a bagel with cream cheese and a peach Danish for breakfast at the office. Just because your peers and bosses do it, it doesn't mean *you* should.

GI Joe Mindset: Remember you are not like everyone, you are not average, so don't treat yourself as one. Many people are happy living on welfare and making ends meet every month, but that doesn't mean you have to. So never use people who are failing as role models; never follow a loser and expect victories. History is made by those who think differently. *Highest goals are most often achieved by those who dare go against all odds and think outside the box.*

BELIEF #3

Average Joe Brain: "You deserve that piece of cake," your spouse tells you. "You worked out so hard today, come on and have a piece of cake with me." Your brain says *"It's true, you deserve it!"* and you end up indulging everyday, every week. You then find yourself after months of hard gym work still overweight, with high cholesterol and not much progress to show for it.

GI Joe Mindset: Many people walk around with a sense of entitlement. But the truth is, and you will probably agree with me, that anything worthwhile that you have achieved in life has required hard work and commitment – whether it was to raise a family, get a college degree, have a savings account and retirement plan, etc. Now why do you think it is any different with your health? *You must work hard to keep it and commit to your goals.* If there is something you deserve, it is to feel great, strong and healthy, and have control over your food choices. This is real power.

BELIEF #4

Average Joe Brain: *"I can't!",* "I can't run a mile," "I can't lose weight," "I can't eat healthy," "I can't keep a food journal." These are all big fat excuses that are not only lies, but sadly, can become a reality for that person. The scary part about this is that the more you use them, the more they will become part of your core beliefs, and trust me, you don't want that, because it will set you up for failure.

GI Joe mindset: This was a phrase I kept on repeating to myself every time I heard the wake up siren go off that summer in Military Camp. Not only do I actually wake up at 5:00 a.m. every day now (and its not that I couldn't), but I wasn't used to it. So, instead of saying "I can't," use words like "I'm not used to it" or "I haven't done it before but today is the day I will." That's how a soldier thinks. *Just because its a lonely road doesn't mean it can't be traveled.*

BELIEF #5

Average Joe Brain: *"I will do it later."* Taking action now has tremendous creative power. Leaving things for later – tomorrow, next week, next year – has tremendous destructive power. The average person procrastinates, never starts exercising, sets goals that never get reached, all because when it comes to taking action, they say *"I will do it later."*

GI Joe Mindset: Some people only eat the crumbs of what others leave. What this means is that some people take actions today while others live off the leftovers. Reaching fitness and health goals is a journey, and a journey consist of steps. Steps have to be taken and what better moment to take them than now. As you start taking steps, actions and decisions geared toward your goals, an overwhelming sense of power and satisfaction will come over you and help you keep taking further steps of progress. *As one sage said, "motion creates motion."*

The 7 days at Military Summer Camp were over before I knew it. I still felt like crying but not out of desperation. It was from happiness and joy, because I had become someone I wanted to become. I became a strong young person who was not afraid to take action and lead others to success. I still weighed 150 pounds, but inside I felt like a 200 pound soldier who could not be defeated – one who was ready to take on any goal or mission. **I had traded my 'average Joe Brain' for a new "G I Joe Mindset."**

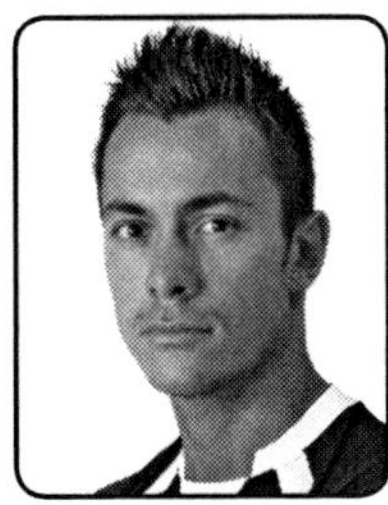

ABOUT JP

Giampiero "JP" Montanari, son of immigrants, and an immigrant himself, discovered at a very early age that any achievement in life requires: Passion, Effort and Sacrifice. These three words have become part of his character not only as a person but as a professional in the fitness and wellness field.

Giampiero "JP" Montanari is Miami's Hispanic Celebrity Trainer, founder of **Coached Fitness** in Hallandale Beach, Fl, and creator of the "90 Day Journey To Your Best Shape Ever". This is a revolutionary system, designed for the average person, to transform your body in just 90 days. Clients receive a 3-phase nutrition plan, specially designed, supplement options, a detailed fitness guide, a calendar to track your progress, online trainer support, Fitness Test, and much more. JP, Your Personal Coach, will keep you engaged every step of the way, and you won't believe your results! His program will enable you to lose those unwanted pounds, gain muscle tone, and improve your overall health and appearance.

He resides in Aventura, FL with his beautiful wife, Claudia.

In pursing a career in the field of health, nutrition and fitness, JP has begun cultivating a diverse educational foundation.

- Sports Nutritionist
- Personal Training Certification by National Academy of Sports Medicine (NASM)
- Completion of the Heartsaver AED (CPR/AED) program by the American Heart Association
- Featured on Channel 7 South Florida
- Weekly TV Fitness Segment on "TDA" Univision reaching all the United States
- Weekly TV Fitness Segment for Venevision International.
- Weekly Radio Fitness Segment on CVC Radio reaching all South America and Europe
- Featured on Miami Local 10 News
- Featured on Almavision TV
- Featured on Renacer Magazine
- Featured on WQBA Radio
- Has help 1000's of people reach their fitness goals thru his services and health tips in Magazines, Radio Shows and Local News

CHAPTER 4

FROM THE BENCH PRESS TO THE BOARD ROOM

– SIX PRINCIPLES USED BY CORPORATE EXECUTIVES THAT CAN HELP YOU REACH YOUR FITNESS GOALS

BY TONY MASLAN, CSCS

Personal training, by its nature, is a luxury. It would be great if everyone could have their very own fitness coach, but the reality is that not everyone can afford to do so. In the 16+ years I have been involved in the fitness industry, I have had the opportunity to work with hundreds of people, and many of them were either business owners or held executive-level positions within their company. As I watch them improve their fitness levels and overall health, I noticed several things that most of these successful business professionals had in common beyond the corporate world. They apply many of the same principles used to building and running a successful company to their fitness programs.

Danny has been a client of mine for over 10 years. He is the CEO of a local company and is someone who I greatly respect. He has run a marathon and maintains a very healthy body weight, body-fat percentage and overall fitness level. During this time that Danny has worked with me, a couple of things stand out: (i) He has done two to three workouts each week with me, every week (with the exception of when he is out of town), for ten years. He has not "taken a break" for a few months here and there. Even when I was gone for ten months with my Marine Corps Reserve unit to Iraq in 2004, Danny still worked out with one of my trainers. (ii) His workouts have taken place between 5:00 am and 6:30 am the entire time. We don't go some mornings, some lunchtimes, some evenings. We are consistent.

As I have worked with Danny and other business executives, these are the commonalities I have found in their programs that have contributed to their ability to achieve a high rate of success in business and in fitness.

1. YOU HAVE TO KNOW WHERE YOU ARE GOING.

When you are planning your fitness program, just like when you are planning your business, you have to have a goal. You need to have both short-term and long-term goals. First determine what your long-term vision is for your fitness program. This vision may change a little bit over time, and that is ok, but you must have an initial picture of what you want to accomplish. For long-term vision, I recommend focusing on things that have to do with your overall health: a healthy body weight and body-fat level, healthy blood pressure, good levels of cholesterol, avoidance of injuries, and general "well-being". I don't recommend that your long-term fitness vision is a specific event or number. For example: run a marathon, bench press 250 pounds, etc. The reason for this is that once you bench press 250 or run your marathon, then what? Are you going to quit? Are you done? I hope not.

With a business, for example, you wouldn't necessarily set a long-term vision to simply gross $1 million in a year. You would probably set it to consistently gross over $1 million dollars with increasing profit margins over time and steadily increasing market share.

Once you have your long-term vision, set short-term goals. These are best done in quarterly, semi-annual, or annual increments depending on the goal. This is where bench pressing 250 or running a marathon fit in – AS LONG AS they are congruent with your long-term vision as well.

Once you have determined your short-term goals and your long-term vision, WRITE THEM DOWN! If you don't write them down, odds are they won't happen.

2. ASSEMBLE THE RIGHT TEAM TO HELP YOU ACHIEVE YOUR GOALS.

In business, I have heard it said that, "if you are the smartest person on your team in every aspect of the organization, you are in trouble." As a CEO you aren't expected to do the accounting, scheduling, marketing, IT work, hiring, new employee orientations, etc. You assemble a team of competent professionals to work within their area of expertise, ultimately leading to a successful organization.

The same approach can be taken with health and fitness. You will not achieve the best results possible if you rely on yourself for your strength training, cardiovascular conditioning, nutritional guidance, massage therapy, chiropractic care and all the other components that go into achieving the long-term fitness vision. A team of professionals including a personal trainer, nutritional counselor or dietician, massage therapist, chiropractor and medical doctor are all essential components of the "health team" that will give you the best chance of achieving that long-term objective.

3. YOUR ACTIVITIES MUST BE CONGRUENT WITH YOUR SHORT-TERM GOALS AND LONG-TERM VISION.

The One Minute Manager by Kenneth Blanchard and Spencer Johnson put it best:

"Look at your goals. Look at your behavior. Does your behavior match your goals?"

In business, if you want to increase sales by 10% over the next quarter, you wouldn't expect that to happen if you went two weeks without scheduling any sales calls or appointments. Similarly, if your fitness goal was to lose weight and decrease body-fat, you aren't going to get that done if you are finishing each dinner with a piece of cake or leaving the gym after your workout and heading out to eat a pizza and drink a couple of pitchers of beer. Those activities are not congruent with your goal.

This doesn't necessarily mean that the activity or exercise that you eliminate is not a "good" one. It just means that it is not moving you towards your goal. For example, if your short-term goal is to increase your bench press to 250 pounds, I would not recommend marathon training at the same time. It doesn't mean that training for a marathon is a "bad thing" it just doesn't go along with your primary short-term objective.

There is an exception that I make to this rule. If there is an activity that my client really enjoys doing, I don't eliminate it completely. For example, if I have a client who loves to get out and run for a couple of hours, using that time as stress relief or whatever, I continue to work that in. I believe it is important to have activities that we actually look forward to and enjoy doing, even if they may not be a perfect fit for our primary objective as long as we take them into account when planning the training program and setting a timeline to achieve the goal.

4. DON'T "MAJOR IN THE MINOR THINGS".

CEO's don't spend their time doing "minimum wage" work. As a business owner or corporate executive, you spend your time working on the things that deliver the most return for the time you put into them. We take the same approach when planning our training programs. We don't spend much time doing isolation exercises such as triceps kickbacks or concentration curls. That doesn't mean that isolation exercises are "bad" or not worth doing ever, they just play a minimal role in our programs. Our clients have other things they would prefer to spend their time on during the day, so we don't keep them in the gym for 2 hours each workout. We make sure that we are as efficient and effective as possible with our workouts – to make sure that we accomplish our objectives in the minimum amount of time possible. In order to do this, our programs consist primarily of compound movements that work more than one muscle group at the same time.

Leg training for our clients starts with squat variations. Everyone does some form of squat. We use overhead squats, front squats, goblet squats, box squats, the traditional barbell squat and more, but EVERYBODY squats. We also include dead-lift variations. After squats and dead-lifts, other leg exercises are a bonus. We still like to focus on multi-joint movements such as lunges and 'step ups' instead of extensions and curls as much as possible.

Upper body training focuses on horizontal pressing and pulling, and vertical pressing and pulling. I'm a big believer in bodyweight exercises, starting with pushups, pull-up variations and body-weight rows. Doing exercises that move your body through space, as opposed to something on a machine, deliver a much higher return and carry-over to your everyday activities.

Moving beyond the bodyweight movements, we use both barbells and dumbbells (as well as the occasional kettlebell), for our horizontal and vertical pressing and some of the horizontal pulling. We do incorporate the lats 'pulldown' machine using different grips for our vertical pulling movements.

For our cardiovascular training we prefer short duration, higher intensity work. We have found that we can get much better results using interval type training (example: jump rope for 1 minute, rest for 30 seconds, repeat 6-10 times) than long, slow, drawn out cardio (example: an hour-long walk on the treadmill). There is a limited amount of time during the day that our clients want to devote to exercise, so we prefer to increase the intensity (speed, incline, resistance) as our client progresses, rather than make them stay on the treadmill, bike or elliptical longer.

5. DOCUMENT AND TRACK EVERYTHING!

This final principal is what separates those who achieve a "good" level of success from those who achieve "great" results. In a business, you want to track progress as much as possible. You always need to "know your numbers". You need to know how much you spent on advertising last month and what your ROI (return on investment) was for those dollars spent. This helps you determine whether or not to use the same marketing program or make adjustments. You have to know what money is going out and where you can cut expenses. The same is true for your fitness program.

A food journal is an absolute must, especially for anyone wanting to lose weight. The more detailed you can be, the better. At a minimum, you need to be able to look at your journal and see everything that you had to eat and drink throughout the day. If you are able to, also track the protein, carbohydrates, fat and calories in what you consume. If you are putting everything that you eat and drink on paper, it is much easier to determine what adjustments you need to make if you are not progressing towards your goal as quickly as you would like. If you don't have a journal, then you are just guessing. Keeping a food journal also makes you think twice before you eat something that doesn't fit in your plan. It has an even more significant impact if you have a personal trainer or nutritional counselor who is going to be looking at that food journal.

A training journal is essential for long-term success as well. First, it is a good way to affirm that what you are doing is moving you the right direction. If one of your goals is to improve your upper body strength, if your journal shows that you could do 5 pushups when you started your program and on your last journal entry you did 20, you know that what you are doing is helping you achieve your objective. This also allows you to repeat phases of training that you feel were especially effective. You can see on paper exactly what you did and in what order.

You can get better without journaling, but you will greatly underachieve.

6. HAVE SOMEONE KEEP YOU ACCOUNTABLE.

We all do better when we are held accountable by someone else. A CEO is accountable to the president of the company and/or the board of directors. Business owners are often accountable to their shareholders. If you have a personal trainer or fitness coach keeping you accountable for your program, you greatly increase your chance of success.

Remember, success leaves clues. Look at the people around you. If you know someone who is successful in business or athletics, you can probably learn something from them that will help you achieve a higher level of success – whether it is with your fitness program or in other areas of life. I hope that these principles I have shared with you help put you on the path to accomplishing your fitness goals more efficiently and effectively.

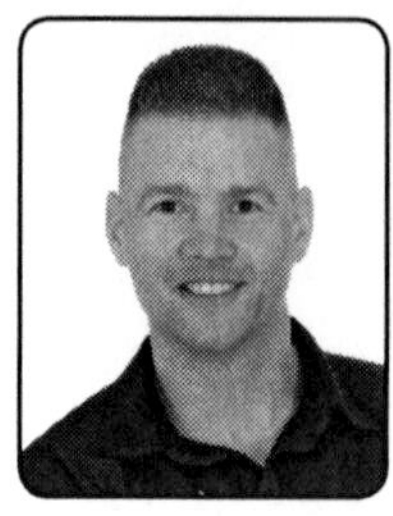

ABOUT TONY

Tony Maslan is a Certified Strength and Conditioning Specialist and the owner of Custom Fit Personal Training in Evansville, Indiana. He specializes in helping people achieve maximum fitness and weight loss results in minimum time, and in helping companies achieve actual measurable results with their wellness programs.

Tony has been in the fitness industry for over 16 years. He started Custom Fit in 2005, after returning from Iraq where he served as an infantry squad leader with the United States Marine Corps Reserves. Custom Fit has quickly become the premier private training company in the tri-state area.

Tony and his wife Chrissie have 4 children: Owen, Nikolas, Maggie and Joshua.

Tony is available for corporate seminars as well as private fitness coaching. To find out how Tony can help you or your company, you can contact him at 812-437-2378 or by email at: tmaslan@cfpt.us You can get more information on Custom Fit Personal Training at: www.EvansvillePersonalTraining.com

CHAPTER 5

HOW TO ENHANCE FITNESS, HEALTH, AND FAT LOSS BY OPTIMIZING YOUR SLEEP

BY DOUG JACKSON, M.ED., CSCS

Exercise and nutrition are clearly important to health and fitness, but the importance of getting enough sleep has been underappreciated. Most people go to trainers and get "worked out". Maybe they'll get on a solid nutrition plan. But most fitness professionals are still not coaching their clients enough on the importance of optimizing their sleep. Assuming that you are already on a scientifically-sound fitness and nutrition program, adequate sleep might just be the piece of the puzzle that you have been missing. As the Centers for Disease Control and Prevention states on its website, "sleep is not a luxury – it is a necessity – and should be thought of as a *vital sign* of good health."

Let me share a story with you. It takes place before my move to sunny South Florida during my junior year at Bowling Green State University in Ohio. In January of that year, at the start of the second semester, I was given a BIG opportunity to develop and grow a personal training program at the university. I was pretty pumped.

At the same time, I was still taking classes, and one of the "easier" classes that semester focused on wellness and stress management. As part of the class, we had to monitor overall fitness indicators including our "resting heart rate". During the first week of class, my resting heart rate was approximately 55 beats per minute. That indicated that my health and fitness were very good.

Throughout the semester, I burned the candle at both ends, thinking that I was invincible. In addition to my class schedule, workout schedule, and the development of the university's new personal training program, I was working my regular job to pay the bills. That meant I wasn't getting much sleep during the week. Then on weekends, I was going out and doing the things most juniors in college do – staying up late and partying a bit too hard.

To fit it all in, I was drinking coffee and energy drinks like a madman and felt like I needed large amounts of caffeine to get me through the day. Throughout the semester, my resting heart rate was increasing by 5-10 beats per month and by the end of the semester, it was hovering around 85 or so. I'm not sure if that means much to you, but someone with a resting heart rate of 85 is not healthy. And going from a resting heart rate of 55 beats per minute to 85 beats per minute within a sixteen-week period is cause for alarm.

It all crashed down on the Saturday after the semester ended. I woke up that Saturday morning and looked like Rocky Balboa after a fight – my eyes were swollen over and my entire face was bloated. It was a severe case of strep throat combined with mononucleosis all at once. I laid in bed shaking and sweating for days, and lost about fifteen pounds in two weeks. I attribute what happened to running my body 'into the ground' by not getting enough rest, recovery, and sleep.

In the ten years since, I still battle with periods of time that I'm working too much and not getting enough sleep, but I'm more aware of it now. Interestingly, although the story I shared with you was somewhat dramatic, my challenges with lack of sleep now are more similar to what most 'folks' experience. Here's what I find: when I'm not getting enough sleep, my food choices and motivation to exercise begin to suffer, ... and then it's a downward spiral. I can tie periods of increased work and less sleep directly to gaining body fat and losing muscle. Because of the importance of sleep, the quality and quantity of sleep are one of the things that we really focus on with our personal training clients.

Think you're getting enough sleep? That you've learned to get by on less? In general, if you're waking up to an alarm clock, you're not getting enough. If your body didn't need more sleep, you would have woken up on your own own. According to the National Sleep Foundation, 63% of American adults do not get the recommended eight hours of sleep per night. In fact, researchers have found that over the past 40 years, sleep duration has decreased by an average of one to two hours per night in the United States.

The vast majority of adults need somewhere between seven and nine hours of sleep per night. Scientists are finding that your optimal sleep is very individualized. One person may feel their best at seven hours per night, whereas someone else would feel tired with only seven hours of sleep and need nine instead. According to Tony Schwartz in the book *The Way We're Working Isn't Working*, "when researchers test subjects in environments without clocks or windows and ask them to sleep whenever they feel tired, approximately 95% of them sleep between seven and eight hours out of every twenty-four."

To support my premise that sleep is an underappreciated key to short-term fitness improvement and long-term health management, I'll be reviewing the following in this chapter:

- How lack of sleep affects your appetite control and body mass index
- How lack of sleep interferes with weight loss programs
- How lack of sleep impacts workout performance
- How lack of sleep increases the risk of injury during exercise
- How lack of sleep impacts willpower and fitness program adherence
- How lack of sleep affects your immune system

SLEEP, "APPETITE CONTROL", AND BODY MASS INDEX

Inadequate sleep lowers the hormone leptin, and increases the peptide ghrelin. In a study by Spiegel, et al., published in the *Annals of Internal Medicine*, two consecutive days of sleep restriction (four hours of sleep per night), was associated with an 18% decrease in leptin, a hormone which inhibits appetite, and a 28% increase in ghrelin, a peptide which stimulates appetite. These changes were associated with a 24% increase in hunger within the test subjects. These results may explain why other studies have found a consistent link between short sleep durations and increased body mass indexes in subjects.

HOW LACK OF SLEEP INTERFERES WITH WEIGHT LOSS PROGRAMS

A 2010 study published in the *Annals of Internal Medicine* examined whether sleep restriction would impact the results from a reduced-calorie diet. The researchers put all participants on a calorie-restricted diet; they then split the group into two groups that would either sleep 8.5 hours vs. 5.5 hours, respectively. The group which slept 5.5 hours lost 55% less fat than the group who slept 8.5 hours. In addition, the restricted sleep group increased their loss of fat-free body mass by 60%. The take away: lack of sleep not only slowed down fat loss, but also sped up muscle loss.

SLEEP AND ITS IMPACT ON WORKOUT PERFORMANCE

Not getting enough sleep starts to kill your motivation to workout intensely over time. It isn't rocket science, when you are not getting enough sleep, you just don't have the energy you need to push your body really hard. And if you are not exercising intensely, you simply will not make any significant improvements in your fitness level for a sustained period.

SLEEP AND DIETARY WILLPOWER

When you are tired, your ability to make the best food choices is impaired. This happens for a few different reasons. First, your willpower to make good food choices is less strong when you are tired. Second, when you are tired, your body is under stress. Stress makes you crave sugars, fats, and salt – basically all the things you don't want to eat when trying to get in shape and look your best.

SLEEP AND IT'S EFFECT ON INJURY PREVENTION

One of the things you will hear from experienced fitness buffs is that a high preponderance of injuries that they've experienced over the years have occurred when they were not getting adequate rest. Sleep deprivation affects not only optimal muscle functioning, but also mental focus, both of which can lead to injury.

SLEEP AND ITS IMPACT ON FITNESS PROGRAM ADHERENCE

From a behavioral standpoint, to stick with a fitness program, you need to be proactive. And you can't just do it when you feel like it. You can safely bet that when you are in a reactive state, you will not be making the best choices when it comes to sticking with your workout routine. When you are sleep deprived and just trying to get through the day, you can kiss your dreams of a great body and better health goodbye.

SLEEP AND YOUR IMMUNE SYSTEM

Not getting enough sleep lowers your immune system and increases your likelihood of getting sick. Diwakar Balachandran, MD, director of the Sleep Center at the University of Texas M.D. Anderson Cancer Center in Houston states, "A lot of studies show our T-cells go down if we are sleep deprived. And inflammatory cytokines go up. ... This could potentially lead to the greater risk of developing a cold or flu." Bottom line: to get and stay fit, you need to have a strong immune system and this will be supported by getting enough sleep.

FIVE TOP REASONS WE DON'T GET ENOUGH QUALITY SLEEP

1. Too much caffeine – too late in the day
2. Too much emotional stress
3. Too much artificial light and television before bed
4. Taking on too many projects. Learn to say "no".
5. Not getting in enough exercise and balanced meals.

EIGHT STRATEGIES FOR IMPROVED SLEEP

1. Create a dark and quiet sleep environment (turn the TV and computer off).
2. Aim to keep a regular sleep schedule.
3. Avoid caffeine after 4:00 pm. If you are up for the challenge, consider eliminating it completely.
4. Write down your "to-do" list each night before bed to enhance your ability to relax and clear your mind.
5. Do not drink alcohol to unwind in the evenings.
6. Avoid late evening exercise if you notice that it disrupts your sleep quality or quantity.
7. Make a real commitment to getting in bed and turning off the lights at a time that will allow you to get a full eight hours of sleep.
8. If you have trouble falling asleep, try deep breathing and progressive relaxation techniques.

CONCLUSION

To make sleep a key part of your fitness and performance program, you need to accept the importance of sleep and commit to quality sleep habits. There is no question that getting enough sleep is an important part of a complete health and fitness plan. As Eve Van Cauter of the University of Chicago Medical Center states, "Lack of sleep disrupts every physiologic function in the body. We have nothing in our biology that allows us to adapt to this behavior." I encourage you to be aware of your sleep habits and work toward improving your sleep patterns with the same dedication that you focus on your fitness and nutrition program.

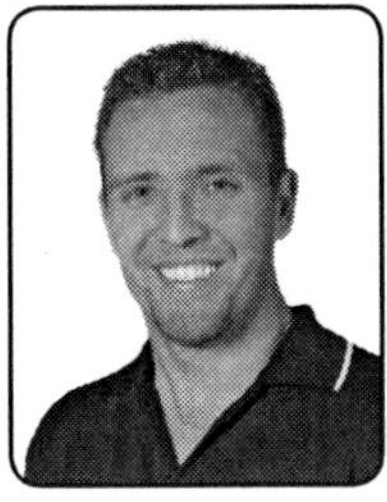

ABOUT DOUG

Doug Jackson, M.Ed., CSCS, is owner of the Personal Fitness Advantage personal training studio in Plantation, Florida. One of the premier personal trainers in the United States, he is also a fitness author who focuses on peak performance psychology, stress physiology, and metabolism. He trains an exclusive group of South Florida's most influential entrepreneurs, medical professionals, and corporate leaders. He is driven by a mission "to help as many people as possible enjoy the vast benefits of fitness".

Doug holds a Bachelor's degree as an Exercise Specialist and a Master's degree in Kinesiology with an emphasis in Exercise Psychology. He is active in the fitness industry's professional associations including the National Strength and Conditioning Association and the American College of Sports Medicine. Doug has been an astute practitioner of physical conditioning techniques for the last eleven years, and in the process has helped hundreds of people achieve a level of fitness that they had only dreamed of attaining.

Considered one of the fitness industry's most prolific writers, he has co-authored the unique *Family Fit Plan*, authored his *Fitness Now and Forever* program, and published in the prestigious *Strength and Conditioning Journal.* You can get more information about Personal Fitness Advantage, receive Doug's leading fitness newsletter, and contact Doug at www.PersonalFitnessAdvantage.com

CHAPTER 6

WHAT EXERCISE IS BEST?

— ONLY *YOU* KNOW THE ANSWER

BY CHRIS WEIGEL

How is it that the United States, arguably the most powerful country in the world, sees its population become fatter and more unhealthy… year after year after year??? How can a nation so fat not prioritize exercise? Note that 63.1% of adults in the U.S. were either overweight or obese in 2009[1]. Are we lazy people? Do we have too many other priorities? What's our excuse? It's not like we're not 'in the know' about how exercise contributes to good health. Obesity, diabetes and other problems that we can avoid with exercise are constantly in the news. Do you have an excuse?

It's my hope that you're already one of the 31% of adults who exercise moderately for 30 minutes five times a week, or vigorously for 20 minutes three times a week[2]. You realize the benefits of exercise and make it a priority because you care about yourself enough to do so. The key for you then is to find a way to exercise that motivates you and that you'll do regularly…for the rest of your life! This shouldn't be difficult considering your desire to exercise and the many different options available today. Honestly, with so many different outlets for exercise readily available, you can literally determine what type of movement makes you feel good – hiking, sports, stretching, dancing, etc. – and find a local group, class or video that facilitates your desires.

If you're not one of the 31%, I bet you're not one of the 40% of the population who don't do squat (pardon the pun) when it comes to exercise.[2] As much as I'd love to speak a few choice words into those peoples' ears, they're probably not the ones reading this book at the moment. Why? Because when it comes to exercise they just don't care. And guess what? That's their prerogative and I respect it. Personally however, I'd rather not be supporting higher healthcare costs because a bunch of people decided not to care for themselves. Don't get me started on that topic. Let's get back to those who care about exercise like you.

If you're not one of the two types of people listed above, you're most likely a 'fence-sitter.' You know you need to exercise. Sometimes you do… for a little while. You just can't seem to find the time, stay motivated, get results or all of the above. I understand and I feel your pain. Even as a health & fitness professional I feel your pain. Everyone, myself included, has competing priorities with exercise. We all wish we loved every minute of strenuous exercise and saw results on a daily basis. But, this just isn't reality. That's why I'm writing this chapter. This chapter is dedicated to the 'fence-sitters' and the regular exercisers alike, because at any given time we all need to find a way to ENJOY exercise and see RESULTS. When it comes to exercise, there is no one-size-fits-all approach to *what* you should do or *where* you should do it. That said, the following three questions will help you figure out which options are best for you:

QUESTION #1

DO YOU GENERALLY LIKE TO BE WITH OTHER PEOPLE, OR ARE YOU MORE OF AN INTROVERT?

Either is fine. While social butterflies may benefit from some introspective time alone (just like the introvert may benefit from time spent with others), the goal here is to get you physically active, not to change your psychological make-up.

If you like to be with other people, you'll probably be well suited to join a health club or gym-type facility. Here you'll find lots of like-minded people trying to utilize exercise to accomplish goals similar to yours. You may feel a little intimidated or overwhelmed at first, but if the fitness center has a friendly staff and good programming to boot, you should be introduced to the facility at a fairly comfortable pace. If you feel a bit lost, ask the staff for help. You'll be a "gym rat" in no time.

Unfortunately, there are plenty of these facilities that do little more than sell you a membership card and leave you to figure things out on your own. If you get that vibe from your initial tour of the facility, don't sign-up to run on their treadmill...RUN IN THE OTHER DIRECTION!!! There are many different types of fitness centers. Find the one you feel comfortable with. One more tip: make sure it's convenient; preferably within a ten minute drive-time. Typically, you'll discontinue the use of a fitness facility if the location isn't convenient for you.

If you're more of an introvert, it's no excuse to hole up in your house and not exercise. You've got lots of great options. Here's an easy one: go for a walk around your neighborhood. You could probably benefit from the fresh air alone. Of course, depending on where you live, you might have a few obstacles in your way (i.e., snow, rain, dogs, and hoodlums). Therefore, it's always good to have an indoor option. With so many television fitness shows and videos now available, it's pretty easy to find a type of exercise you'll enjoy doing indoors. Interactive fitness video options such as the Nintendo Wii can be especially entertaining and have a wide selection of games and instructional videos that you can move your body to. I still wouldn't necessarily rule out participating at a fitness center, however, where you can always put your headphones on and tune everyone else out.

QUESTION #2
WHAT IS YOUR CURRENT FITNESS LEVEL?

If you're a beginner or novice, meaning you're anywhere between having never exercised and having done a little walking or simple cardio, don't worry. Exercise can be made as easy as needed and the intensity increased as you adapt. Progression is key. Let your walk turn into a longer walk. Let your longer walk turn into a jog. Let your jog turn into sprint intervals. If you're lifting weights, progress by using more weight or doing more reps. As a beginner or novice, you're well suited to begin exercising with just your body-weight (i.e., calisthenics). If you search the web for "calisthenics" or "body-weight exercises" you'll find plenty of options to do in your own home. Many of the websites will have videos of the exercises to help you perform the exercise properly. Just don't do too much too fast. It's better to take a slow, yet steady approach to progression. Just remember, "A little, often, over the long haul!"

Check out a Certified Personal Trainer at a nearby fitness facility if you're looking for a more individualistic and time-efficient approach to exercise. A good trainer will make a quick assessment of what you should or shouldn't do to reach your goals as quickly as possible and without injury. The last thing you want when starting an exercise routine is to injure yourself. Injuries can set back your progress and squash your motivation. What exercises suit you best and how to perform them is not inherent knowledge. Knowing the body and what will benefit it is a deep and ever-changing field of study. The designation "Personal Trainer" is now a degree at some universities. You wouldn't do your own electrical work at home without being certain about what you were doing, right? The same goes for working on your body. It's best to get professional direction. This advice holds true regardless of one's fitness level.

Even the more advanced exercise participant will benefit from professional guidance, including the professional athlete. A specific, progressive program is necessary for anyone who is looking to take their training to a higher level. Such a program isn't necessary if you're looking to maintain your current fitness level, but it can still be beneficial in an effort to keep exercise new, interesting and fun. I've found that most people who continue to do the same exercises, workout after workout, either quit eventually because of boredom, or worse yet, develop overuse injuries from repeating the same movements over and over... and over. Being honest about your starting point is key, but so is knowing where you want to go. This brings me to my last question:

QUESTION #3
WHAT IS YOUR GOAL?

Asking yourself this question will go a long way towards determining what type of exercise is best for you. Do you want to lose weight or build muscle? Are you not as nimble as you used to be, or perhaps in pain? Are you looking to improve your performance in a particular sport? Is health or longevity your primary focus? These questions and others are critical to ask yourself so as to determine the type of exercise that will accomplish your goal(s).

It's beyond the scope of this chapter to address all the different types of exercise related to cardiovascular conditioning, strength training, flexibility and more specific categories related to health and fitness. However, I want to mention a few critical, yet oftentimes overlooked, options.

If you would like to exercise but are reluctant because of current aches and pains in your muscles or joints, seek a "Corrective Exercise Specialist" or highly skilled massage therapist who can perform a hands-on assessment that will help determine what type(s) of exercise will not only alleviate your pains, but also help you to attain your goal(s). If weight loss is your focus with exercise, and you want a little guidance, make sure the source of your guidance recognizes the importance of a proper diet. While I'm a HUGE proponent of exercise, there's no substitute for a healthy diet. Lastly, if you're a well-seasoned gym-rat or athlete looking to reach the next goal you've set for yourself, seek someone who is really 'in the know.' Don't rely on the news stand magazines with sexy headlines. You need to find a professional with a background in what YOU aim to achieve.

Overall, the sincerest advice I can give you is to realize that when it comes to 'what is best for you,' you must do your own research and become your own expert. There are so many books, websites, infomercials, "experts" and other sources of opinion out there to influence you that it's difficult to decipher what is truth and what is fiction. However, if your goal is a high enough priority in your life, you will spend the necessary time needed to determine 'what is best for you.' Become your own expert just as you would when buying a car, getting a loan or determining what's in fashion.

Bottom-line: take charge of your own health and well-being, and realize that you're unique – one-size-does-not-fit-all. Spend the necessary time to decipher *what is best for YOU*; seek and work with a health and fitness professional that understands YOU; focus on what YOU aim to accomplish, and find a way to make exercise fun. No matter what your age, no matter what your fitness level…you can always attain a higher level of health and fitness by seeking the best exercise option for YOU!

---

(1) Gallup-Healthways Well-Being Index 2009

(2) The National Health Interview Survey

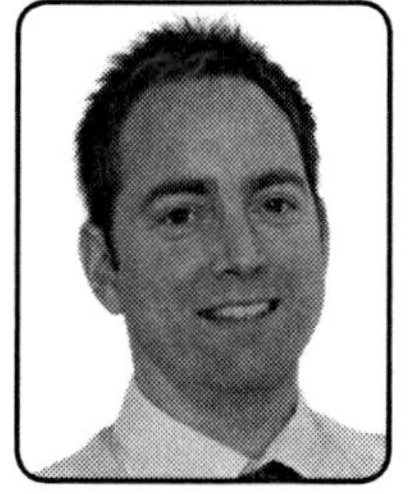

ABOUT CHRIS

Before Chris' formal education in health and fitness began, he was convinced that he would be happy making a living if he simply pursued what he loved to do – hang out in the gym and talk to other people about working out, eating right and feeling good.

With that in mind, Chris Weigel dedicated his collegiate years (1993-97) at Winona State University to earning a Bachelor of Science degree in Exercise Science, conducting extensive research and developing sport-specific programs for the Rochester Mayo Clinic, working various positions at local health clubs, and becoming certified through the National Strength & Conditioning Association as a Personal Trainer and Strength & Conditioning Specialist. Armed with this knowledge, he moved to Dallas, Texas to pursue his desire to help others as a personal trainer.

He quickly broke sales records for the Fitness Factory club chain in Dallas before incorporating his own athletic development company in 2000 – All-Star Development Systems, Inc. Chris earned certifications as a C.H.E.K - Certified Golf Biomechanic and U.S.A.T.F.- Certified Level I Track & Field Coach during this time, while managing a team of coaches who trained local athletes at their respective training facilities.

In 2002, Chris opened his first gym-type facility – Fit-Zone – where he continued to work with athletes and the general public alike. For five years he worked successfully as an owner and personal trainer, helping hundreds find success with fitness. He collected numerous other certifications during this time; becoming a C.H.E.K- Certified Level II Practitioner, C.H.E.K- Certified Level II Nutrition & Lifestyle Coach, and HealthExcel - Certified Metabolic Typing Advisor. This background helped Chris develop a holistic practice which addressed peoples' emotional, mental and spiritual roadblocks to attaining their health and fitness goals.

Chris would next parlay this success into his next business venture in 2010 – Clairevista Vitality Club. This is what he now pours his passion for health and fitness into – managing most aspects of a club well-diversified in its approach and offerings. Chris and his team of specialists believe that there is no one-size-fits-all approach to exercise, nutrition or any other aspect of leading a fit and healthy lifestyle. For this reason, Chris' team works together and provides a wide array of programming options to meet their member's needs. This individualized yet holistic approach provides club members real solutions for getting fit, maintaining great health and living happier lives.

CHAPTER 7

FOUR LESSONS THAT WILL SHAPE THE MOST POWERFUL FAT-LOSS SUCCESS TOOL YOU OWN

BY CLINT BARR

When you have to make a choice and don't make it, that is in itself a choice.
~ William James

It seems minor; in fact, most of the time you aren't even consciously aware of it. Day-in, day-out the secret to successfully achieving your fat loss goals is right there in front of you. It's in the tiny, seemingly insignificant decisions you make every day. But so many times you fail to recognize the "weight" your choices bear on the outcome of your success.

I know exactly what that is like, because as a struggling entrepreneur I failed to see that my success was directly related to the choices I was making. What's more, I thought I made a decision to be a business owner where in fact I actually just owned a job. Much in the same way, you decide to lose weight but never own up to the fact that you still haven't made the transition from decision to implementation. You simply lack the understanding of the most powerful tool you possess that will guarantee your success…your *choices*.

When I first opened my personal training business, I aspired to be the best personal training business in my town. I was going to grow and multiply incessantly, or so I thought. So, I made the decision to open my business, but never *really* made the correct choices to be called a business owner. I started out, just me training clients in a 500 square foot room with minimal equipment, and it wasn't long until my schedule was full. That's when I became blind to the decisions I was making for the business that progressively dug me a deeper and deeper hole.

I didn't really have a clear picture of what I wanted the business to look like, and that influenced how I took on clientele. As time went on the business did grow, but eventually it would hit a limit at which I could no longer function optimally. I was a 'one man show' after all, and therein lay the problem. With no clear vision of how I saw my business going forward, it clouded my judgment and I began to believe that no one was capable of training the clients the way I was training them (which is obviously a false belief system and mindset to have as a business owner.)

So as time went on, I got sucked further and further into working "in" the business, which depleted my ability to effectively work "on" the business, thus bringing any kind of healthy growth to a complete stand still. I had become my own worst enemy in the battle to achieve my goal of being the best personal training business in my town. Don't get me wrong, I think I'm a great personal trainer, but my goal was to be the best personal training *business*. It wasn't that I didn't want to be the best, I just couldn't realize the significance of my choices; choices that caused more harm than good – not just in the growth of the business but in my personal life as well.

From 4 a.m. to 7 p.m. Monday through Friday I worked non-stop without any breaks. There was no time for my workouts, nor did I have time to eat lunch. I would come home around 7:30 p.m. only to work on the administrative things that needed to be done to keep the business moving, which resulted in not eating dinner on most nights. Saturdays consisted of six hours of training clients followed by a few hours of drawing up workout plans and doing some writing for my blog. After only sleeping about 5 hours a night for more than a year, and not taking care of myself physically, nutritionally, or spiritually, I reached a breaking point.

As you can imagine, there wasn't much room left for investing in my own physical fitness and well-being, nor my marriage. My personal life spun out of control and ultimately led to poor physical health, and being just one phone call away from being served with divorce papers. Not exactly what I had in mind when I opened my doors more than a year before. Luckily, I recognized my downfall before it was too late, and I had a business coach that helped me get back on the right track and focused on the goal I initially made for myself and my business. In just over a year I pulled myself out of that hole and I now have a thriving business with 5 wonderful employees, who give me the freedom and ability to work 100% on the business, driving it toward being the best personal training business in my town.

You're probably scratching your head right about now asking, *what in the world does that have to do with reaching your fat loss goal,* right? Well, remember I told you that the most powerful tool you possess that guarantees success is choice. And there are four very important lessons that you can learn from my story that will help you recognize and make the correct choices once you make the decision to lose weight and keep it off for good.

LESSON #1
HAVE A CLEAR VISION

This is where I made my first mistake as a business owner. I didn't *really* know what I wanted the business to look like. If you don't have a detailed image (goal) of exactly what you want your body to look like, realistically of course, then you'll never be able to effectively make the proper decisions required to achieve that goal. So you need to sit down and really think about what you want in terms of your body weight, the size of clothes you want to fit into, and how you want to look. You need to make it so clear, so vivid and so detailed that you could actually touch it. Let it burn into your mind and make it stick. I'm not going to give a lesson on goal setting, that's a book chapter by itself, but you should definitely write down the goals you have for yourself, show them to someone, set a deadline for achieving them, and post them where you'll be reminded of them on a daily basis.

The vision is vital to your success, because it will govern the choices you make on a daily basis. If you have a burning desire to make your vision a reality, then your choices will be in line with those goals. It's that simple. But if you never have a clear vision, then your choices are going to be as random as a feather blowing in the wind…never knowing where it will end up.

LESSON #2
CHANGE YOUR BELIEF SYSTEM AND MINDSET

Our choices are also determined by what we believe. As an aspiring personal trainer turned fitness business owner I didn't think anyone else would be capable of training the clients as well as I could. The fact is, once I stripped myself of that false belief system, I found that not only could someone else train the client as well as I could, but in most cases they did it even better. And I'm thankful for that fact. This is an important lesson. You *must* purge any false belief or mindset you've been carrying around your entire life before you will be successful at achieving your body weight goals. Think about it. In defensive driving class, they teach you to look where you want the car to go when you are suddenly breaking violently trying to avoid a collision. If you keep looking at the object you're trying to avoid then you can't see where the safest place to go will be. More often than not, by looking at that object you're trying to avoid you inevitably hit it. How could you possibly make choices that help you reach your goal if your mindset and belief system are always turning you back to the self-sabotaging choices you've made your whole life? You can't.

Believe in yourself. When you have a clear vision and a strong belief system/mindset you become a powerful, self-motivated, goal-achieving machine. You are capable of doing more than you think you can. All you have to do is force yourself to see your own potential. Once you do, making good, healthy choices that directly align to support your goal will become second nature.

LESSON #3
DON'T MAKE EXCUSES

Excuses happen when you don't have a clear vision and you have a poor belief system. When I was working in my business 14-15 hours a day my excuse was nobody will know what these clients need more than me, …and that fed the excuse engine. Things like, *I won't be able to find quality employees* or *I can't trust someone to give these clients the service they deserve.* Think about the excuses you make when it comes to reaching your health and fitness goals. Have you ever said "I don't wake up that early," or "I don't like vegetables," or "___ ___ ___" (you fill in the blanks)? Progress involves change. Sometimes you have to go against what you normally do, because what you normally do on a daily basis is the very thing that is making it hard for you to reach your goal. You can either make excuses or make progress. You can't do both. It's a choice! You choose to go workout, or you don't. You choose to eat a clean, healthy diet, or you don't. It's that simple. So stop making excuses and start making progress. Once you strip away the excuses by choosing to do what is necessary to reach your desired fat-loss goal, the path is suddenly more clear, better lit, and easier to maneuver.

LESSON #4
HAVE SOMEONE HOLD YOU ACCOUNTABLE

You need another person or group of people to know what your goals are in order to be successful. I have friends that I meet with weekly and we talk about life. I need them to hold me accountable in my personal life. I have an awesome team of business coaches and mentors that help me keep my business on track and working toward the goals I have set for it. There are times when I have ideas or thoughts that need to be heard by someone else and repeated back to me so I know whether or not they make sense. You need the same thing.

An accountability partner, or even better, a personal trainer, someone who knows your goals in detail, will help you adhere to making good choices. They'll be there to remind you of the path you have chosen. Accountability is a necessary component in achieving your fat-loss goal and in determining your choices. The simple fact that someone else will know that you did or didn't do what you set out to do will have a profound effect on the way you make decisions.

THE CHOICE TOOL

All too often we tend to forget about the small, seemingly minor, choices that we make hundreds of times a day. We focus more on the major decisions. The truth is… all of our choices have an outcome. More importantly, our choices create a habitual response that lead to a consistent, predictable end result. This means that we determine exactly what we want in life. And it is our decisions (choices) that will develop the outcome we desire. By having a clear vision, a strong belief system, and someone to hold you accountable, you *will* make choices that lead to your desired fat-loss goal.

You can have the body you desire… the only thing holding you back is YOU. It's a choice. Is it going to be hard? ABSOLUTELY! But what things in life are more appreciated and more celebrated than the things for which you worked hard to achieve or accomplish? Nothing! So I ask you... *are you going to make excuses? Or are you going to make progress?*

You decide!

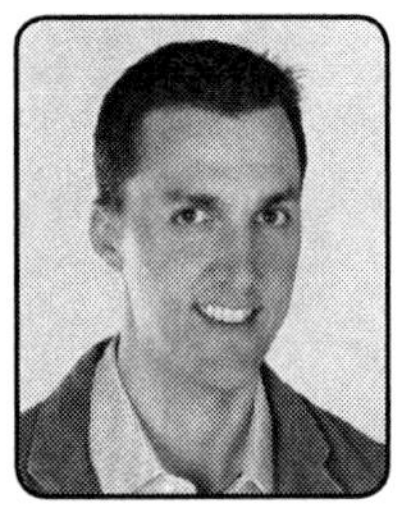

ABOUT CLINT

Clint Barr started *Raising The Barr Fitness* with one thing in mind – to help people learn the truth about lasting weight loss and health, and to help them reach their health and fitness goals. Based out of Ridgeland, MS, *Raising The Barr Fitness* has been dedicated to serving and educating everyone seeking lifelong health and fitness with an unparalleled experience in a fun, challenging environment for the past three years.

Clint and his staff of fitness experts provide the most current and relevant information to their clientele and implement programs that are proven to produce results on a consistent basis. All that is expected of those who work with Clint and his team is that they have a goal to reach, and they are committed and passionate about achieving it.

Clint has a broad range of experiences as a **professional athlete, collegiate strength coach, and personal trainer**. His **passion for strength training and fitness** comes from his background as a competitive baseball player. Clint completed his playing career with the **New York Yankees** organization where he spent two seasons at the A-advanced level in Tampa, Florida.

Prior to playing professionally with the Yankees, Clint received a full athletic scholarship to play at McNeese State University in Lake Charles, Louisiana where he earned a **Bachelor's Degree in Exercise Science**. In addition to a career in athletics, Clint has worked as the strength and conditioning coordinator and graduate assistant baseball coach for Louisiana State University Shreveport (LSUS). During his time at LSUS Clint earned a **Master's Degree in Exercise Science**. He also worked at the USA Olympic Weightlifting Development Center located on the campus of LSUS, which led to appointments at the United States Olympic Training Center in Colorado Springs working for **USA Weightlifting**.

Clint is regularly sought out by the media for his fitness expertise, which he has shared on ABC and NBC affiliates, as well as People Magazine and a host of other local publications in his area.

To learn more about Clint Barr, and how you can receive special reports and other applicable health and fitness strategies from one of the country's top personal trainers and fitness business owners, visit: www.RaisingTheBarrFitness.com.

Clint's photo is courtesy of Robert Smith, www.robertsmithimages.net.

CHAPTER 8

IT'S ABOUT GETTING INTO LIFE!

BY GINNY GRUPP, MS

When I met Beth, she couldn't stand up straight. Well, that's not entirely true. She stood up, but her shoulders were so rounded forward (she is a life-long computer programmer) that her poor posture was taking a good inch or so off of her height (she's just about 6ft. tall). A mother of two high-schoolers, she realized that over the years of focusing on raising her family, and building her computer-based business, she had neglected her own health and body. She was still pretty active, hiking, playing golf, and cross-country skiing when she could squeeze it in; but in addition to the bad posture, she was on blood pressure meds. Meds she did not want to be on for the rest of her life. For Beth, weight loss was not her focus. It would be a nice side effect of working out, but it was not her primary goal.

I met Tina in one of our Boot Camp classes. She joined our program with a goal of getting stronger and keeping up with her super-athletic family. Like Beth, Tina has two high-school-aged daughters. In addition, her husband is a super cross-country skier. Also like Beth, Tina was still somewhat active but wanted to be stronger so she could keep up with the kids and ski with her husband. Weight loss was not her primary goal.

Mark (also a computer wizard), came to me with issues similar to Beth. He had rounded shoulders and he was dealing with back pain and had been on blood pressure meds for well over 10 years. More than anything, Mark wanted to address his overall strength, and he wanted to move without pain. And like both Beth and Tina, weight loss was not his primary goal.

What did all of these folks have in common? They wanted to get into shape, *not* because they wanted to look fabulous in a bathing suit. They wanted to be more fit so that they could get more out of life. What does that mean? It means that when your body is strong, you can do more. When you don't have pain you can enjoy every-day activities. Your body is a tool for making your life better. Life is about living and living to the best of your ability. This is what motivates me, what motivates my clients and can motivate you.

Whether your goal is to be stronger or to lose weight, it doesn't matter. It's not about getting into *shape*, it's about getting into *life*! For me, these words are the difference between success and failure. I know what you're thinking, "… a catch phrase is not what I need. I need real, specific direction. I need to know what the secret is to weight loss and fitness."

Focusing on these few words will give you the tools to create your very own plan to achieve the health and fitness success that you're looking for. You already know how to achieve what you want. I'm going to take you through how to get there with this simple phrase. Remember, It's not about getting into *shape*, it's about getting into *life*!

Take a moment to really think about that phrase and to absorb it. Grab a pen or just find yourself a quiet spot to think and then follow the three simple steps that follow.

In our 24-hour/7day a week, 'go, go, go' lifestyle, quiet time for thought and contemplation is hard to come by. I understand that and I'm asking for five minutes of your time. Now that you're settled in, let's begin:

1. Create your "my life" list. Take a few minutes to write down your life. I don't mean start at birth and write a biography. I mean what do you do now in your life? Work, raise the family, coach the kid's sports team, and then there's shopping, cooking, traveling, whatever. Write it all down. To help with this, just

think about what you do in a typical day and then dump all of that information out of your brain and onto the paper.

2. Rate how well you do each of the things in your life. I'll give you some guidelines to clarify what I'm talking about but it's your rating system, so do with it what you want. For example, your kids are 10 and 12 years old. On your "my life" list, you have coach soccer. How well do you do that? Well, you know the skills, so you rate yourself high for knowing what you're teaching. The kids are learning the skills, high rating for teaching ability. You can't run the length of the soccer field with them during practice. Physical abilities gets "needs improvement." Note what you do well or to the best of your ability and note what might be holding you back from doing your best.

3. Address what's holding you back. For those things that you've rated yourself as not doing particularly well, figure out what you can do to improve those things. If we use the soccer example, what can you do to improve your physical fitness? You could just start running or find a personal trainer to help you work on your cardio capacity and while you're at it, they could work on some strength training with you to improve your overall fitness. Improving your fitness may result in a decrease in your elevated blood pressure, making you healthier – meaning your heart will last longer and you'll be able to see your 10 and 12 year olds grow up and maybe you'll play with their kids some day. Maybe now that you're healthier, you and the family will take an active vacation, improving your relationship with them while decreasing your stress levels.

Once you've completed the above three steps, what you'll have is really a list of goals. In our soccer example, the goal becomes 'improve physical fitness.' Yes, you've set this as a goal before. You may even have "get fit" as a goal right now. The difference is that the goals you come up with by going through this process give you the "why" for achieving your goals. This is your motivation.

You want to improve your fitness level so that you can continue to have a bond with your child. You want to coach her team well so she can enjoy the game. It may be that you need to lose weight to do this job better. Again, what will keep you focused on the long-term achieving of this goal is the "why." Why will achieving this goal improve your life? What long-term pain are you resolving by achieving this goal? Remember, it's not about getting into *shape*, it's about getting into *life*! Creating this new goal and having a tie-in with how this goal will make your life better; this is what makes all the difference.

Anyone can follow a diet and exercise program. There are literally thousands to choose from. And doing a *Google* search for diet and exercise turns up literally millions of options. And they all have one thing in common. Each and every diet, exercise and weight-loss program out there gives you exactly what you ask it for – short-term, immediate results. However, they do not help you to maintain long-term results. Often the entire book is about the plan and there is no information whatsoever about how to transition from "the plan" back into real life. They never tell you what to do once you've completed the plan. They do not help you to get back into your life. They are slapping a band-aid on your problems by helping you to feel good for a few weeks.

It's really not about getting into *shape*, it's about getting into *life*! This is more than just a slogan. For me it is the guiding theme of my life. Whenever I do a public speaking event, I talk to people about what this means.

The first question I always ask my audience is how many of them have been involved in a health and fitness program? Almost every hand in the room goes up.

My next question is, "How many of you would say that your program was successful?" About half of the hands go up.

I then go on to give my definition of a successful program. I define a successful program as one that helps you to reach your goals and then helps you to maintain those goals for the rest of your life. Using that definition of success, I ask the question again, "How many of you would say that your program was successful?" This time only a hand or two will go up and those hands usually belong to my clients.

Why is that? Because the focus of their programs is completely different from the focus of programs like mine. My goal is *not* just to get you into shape. My goal is to help you change your life. I sit down with each of my clients and we talk about their goals for working with us. We talk about their life, what's working and what's not. Then we work together to get them back <u>into</u> their life.

Getting into life means something different to everyone. Only you can decide what is important to you and *why* it's important. And you have to take time to do this. It's not something you can decide without some focused "me" time. Remind yourself that you are that important. Yes, YOU! Not the kids, not your spouse, YOU are important in all of this. Take out your calendar and set aside some time to take a look at what you call your life. Is it everything you want it to be? If not, that's ok.

Write, "It's not about getting into *shape*, it's about getting into *life*!" on the top of your page and follow the three steps I've listed at the beginning of this chapter. Make your list and start taking steps towards achieving your goals today.

The changes you are about to make do not happen overnight. Your life consists of years and years of the good, the bad and the ugly. You probably have developed some great habits and some not-so-great habits over the course of your lifetime. How do you undo the bad habits? … One step at a time.

Beth told me a story when we began working together. When her posture started "going bad," her husband used to tell her to stand up straight. Initially, this was taken as a caring suggestion. After hearing it repeated over and over, however, she asked him to keep his thoughts on the matter to himself. He did and her posture worsened to the point that she was at when she came to see me. About a month after we began working on her posture, she asked him to please start telling her when she wasn't standing up straight again. She had made improvements, and by asking him to point out when she wasn't doing what she should, she had a powerful reinforcement tool helping her to work on this thing that would make her life better.

After a while, she was standing tall consistently, and he stopped commenting on her posture – not because she asked him not to, but because she achieved her goal. That kind of teamwork is what helps her to maintain her improved posture to this day. With the improved posture, she also has a better golf game and her knees don't hurt like they used to. She continues to exercise and maintain her goals because she is getting more out of life.

In just eight weeks, Tina lost 13 pounds and changed the eating habits of her entire family. And, while she will never out-ski her husband or daughter, she now does a much better job of keeping up with them. Last summer, the family went on a bike ride together and she was proud to have kept up with them for the entire ride.

The best question that Tina asked me was about seven weeks into her 8-week program. "What do I do when it's over?" My answer was, "What do you mean, when it's over? What's over?" By the 7-week mark, Tina had successfully changed her eating habits, her family's eating habits and was exercising regularly both on her own and in one of our Boot Camp programs. "You just continue doing what you're doing. You live the new life you've already created for yourself." I could tell by the look in her eyes that she had the "ah-ha" moment. "You're right," she said, "I've already made the changes, I'll just keep doing what I'm doing."

And that's the beauty of it. The changes were so simple – adding more veggies, working on portion control, focusing on strength-building – that she made them without realizing that she had made huge changes in her life. Making small, consistent changes is the key to long-term success.

Mark became a regular at the gym. On any Monday, Wednesday and/or Friday, Mark was there at 2:00 pm. The flexibility in his back got to be so good that his doctor told him that in the entire 12 years they had been seeing each other, his back had never looked so good. He came off of his blood pressure meds for the first time in over a decade. Maintaining his weight and living without pain had seemed like an unreachable dream to Mark when we first met. Today, because he has gained so much life back from working with us, you can still find him at the gym on any given Monday, Wednesday or Friday. He has made his health a priority and nothing stops him from doing what he has to do to maintain what he has achieved. He regularly posts his workouts and his meals on FaceBook. He not only has his "my life" list for himself, he has shared it with his FaceBook family. With no hesitation, he has posted that his health and fitness are the number one priorities in his life. He then enjoys support from his friends and family to help him maintain his life.

You can do it, too. Now that you've reached the end of this chapter, go back to the beginning. Write: "It's not about getting into *shape*, it's about getting into *life*!" at the top of your page. Follow steps 1, 2 and 3.

Then get into *life*!

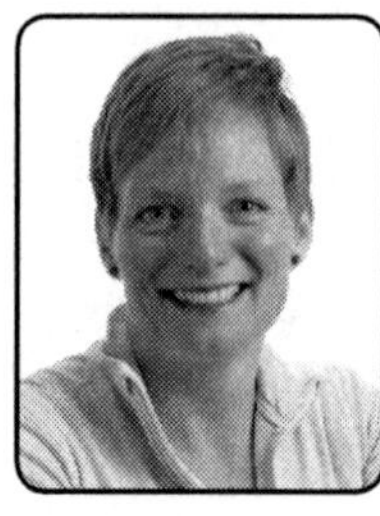

ABOUT GINNY

Born and raised in New York, Ginny Grupp found fitness at twelve years old. That was when she got swept up in the Jane Fonda fitness craze, donned leg warmers and did the "Jane Fonda Workout" 3 times a day in her room. She loved the feeling of strength that came along with the wide variety of exercises and knew somehow, fitness would always be a part of her life.

Off she went to college, where she discovered running and strength training, then to New York City, where she first worked with a personal trainer. Thinking this was a much more fun option than her 9-to-9 job in the financial industry, she eventually left her Wall Street career. Although she had run the NYC marathon and inspired many of her friends and co-workers to add fitness to their lives, she wasn't quite ready to jump from the cubicle to the gym.

Instead, she combined her passion for fitness with a passion for the outdoors and traveled for three years before arriving in Alaska. Here, she found her home. In 2003, she decided that Girdwood, Alaska would be her permanent residence and that it was time to pursue fitness as a full-time career. She became an ACE-certified personal trainer in 2003, continued on to a Master of Science in Exercise Science and Health Promotion, and achieved her Performance Enhancement Specialty certification from the National Academy of Sports Medicine in 2007. She launched AlaskaFit in 2005 and began to grow and expand the business in 2007.

Ginny has worked with hundreds of clients in Alaska and around the United States. She launched AlaskaFit Boot Camps in 2009 and is making health and fitness a priority for Alaskans. Her philosophy is, "It's not about getting into *shape*, it's about getting into *life*!" AlaskaFit's focus for clients is to get them physically fit and active for the simple reason that there is no better way to enjoy life than to feel good. And really, isn't enjoying the ride what life is all about?

CHAPTER 9

FITNESS WITH SOUL

– OFFERING THE FRUITS OF YOUR ACTIONS TO A HIGHER PURPOSE

BY CLAUDIA CASTRO-LEVERETT
& THOMAS LEVERETT

I remember when my wife, at the time girl friend, first told me she was going to start training to run a marathon. We were working our way through college and busy charting our courses to the future. I, of course, being the all-knowing male that I was, immediately told her, "You know the first person who did that fell down and died." ...referring to the urban legend about how marathons started. I could not for the life of me understand why anyone would want to run, especially if no one was chasing them. It was this sort of disdain for exercise that had earned me the extra 35 pounds that clung to me like a baby koala. That same disdain, negativity, and a know-it-all attitude had also landed me in a nice cozy little rut that I was all too happy to stay in. I had, it seemed, slowly begun to stagnate and lose focus.

She on the other hand began to change, grow and, well, pass me up. Running was just the latest thing. She was clearly taking her life in a more defined and purposeful direction, and seeing as how our history went back to Kindergarten, I quickly took notice. At first, I was threatened. If she wanted to run, as many of you other boyfriends and husbands know, it meant *I* was going to have to run. Well not really *had* to, but it would sure be a good idea, so I did.

Years later, working side by side, and trying to make a difference in the world with our daughter, our passion, and our martial arts and fitness studio; we were able to look back on that turning point and see the deep lessons and significance that we had experienced. Life, we had found, was profoundly purposeful and connected in ways that were beyond comprehension, but not beyond reach. Working with high ideals and intuition we had time and time again both together and separately identified our goal, made a plan, and kept ourselves to it. By keeping goals purposeful to our personal growth, we always kept ourselves on our toes, and life was, and is, fulfilling.

While all plans change, there are always some things that remain consistent to the process and the filter through which we learn to view the world and our relationship to it. It starts with understanding that our highest ideals and aspirations lie deep within ourselves, tightly bound to the core of our being, to what we will refer to now as the soul.

MIND, BODY, SOUL.

Mind, Body, Soul. We have heard it recited over and over again in different readings before and we may or may not have thought it was applicable to us. Today it is. The Soul, in its magnitude, houses the totality of our vital, mental, and spiritual energies. It ignites us, connects us and gives us an everlasting reason for being and purpose.

A good way to begin sensing the soul is when the body is tired and the mind has checked out for the day. The soul is that gentle voice that still resides in the background; some say it is the seat of intuition, or the heart of hearts. All of us have the potential to tap into that inner temple and discover our true life's purpose and the path that will get us there. The beauty of our "purpose" is that it is malleable, ever-changing; it takes different shapes and forms at the varied stages in our lives. The soul guides us to ignite the fire that will get us on the path of manifesting that purpose.

WHAT DO I DO NOW?

So you find yourself thinking about all of these "Big" ideas and things that you may or may not have thought about in the past, and you say to yourself, "Ok, but where do I start, and how does this apply to me?" Well, it starts with your intent and desire for what you want for your life and future. Are you happy where you are? Fitness starts in the head with positive thinking, a goal, and a plan. You may be thinking about doing an Ironman, natural child birth, running a marathonor losing 80 lbs. It could be any number of things. The main point is that you are ready for a change and realize that there is more you could be doing for yourself to get fit inside, where it is the most important. Without the proper beliefs about ourselves and what we can truly accomplish, it is nearly impossible to realize our full potential as human beings. The more practice you get setting challenging goals and reaching them, the more you will realize that it is a skill which can be refined and mastered.

You might begin your journey to wellness with your physical and mental body in mind. "I must lose this weight to fit into that dress before my 25th high school reunion!" And at some point the thought changes into, "I've got to stay healthy, so that my kids have a good example to live by." The goal connected to that which lies deeply within – the soul – transforms into something meaningful and relevant.

You must focus on all three aspects: mind, body, and soul in equal measure. If you took one leg from a three-legged stool, it would be unbalanced, inadequately supported and fall. Such are our own attempts at lofty goals and life-long dreams when not supported by the unification of all three supports.

FOUR STEPS TO STAYING CONNECTED, POSITIVE, AND FOCUSED IN YOUR DAILY LIFE

1. FIND STILLNESS

Most of our challenges lie in that we have not calmed ourselves enough to listen to that intuitive power within. Here is one way to begin this process:

Set your alarm clock tomorrow for at least 45 minutes before you need to begin your day. Really. Rise. Wash your face. Grab a cushion and sit facing east where the sun rises. Place your hands palm facing up on your thighs, back straight, close your eyes. Become a witness to your breath. Refrain from letting the mind get involved. Sit without judgment, as if you are simply an observer. From your heart center (right at the sternum), breathe in a beam of gratitude for just that moment. Let it penetrate and fill you. Then allow it to flow out taking all tension and stress away with it. As the next breath comes in, allow an offering to arise from that inner voice, and on the next, connect to that which is your love, your devotion, your inspiration. If you don't know what that means to you yet, don't worry about it. Keep at it, it will come to you.

Take this small amount of time to center and really see what is important in your life. What do you have to be thankful for? What makes you truly happy? What inspires you? This will help to define a purpose that is more in tune with your soul. Stillness, for some, doesn't just mean sitting and meditating. My first most profound and deepest thoughts/meditations, came to me on my long drives, 18 mile long runs, or while camping, just looking at the stars. Stillness helps us reconnect and put greater ideals into perspective.

2. BE PURPOSEFUL

Being purposeful has to do with staying focused on your intentions. What have you decided to do? If you have a serious goal be serious about it. Work on not getting distracted. Being purposeful requires your complete attention on what you are doing. One way of being purposeful in your everyday life is with your conversation. Had I listened to that boyfriend on the couch, I would have never accomplished running three marathons, among other things.

In your conversation, watch out for idle chatter. "What are you doing?"; "What's up?"; "How are you doing?"; "Fine, thanks." If you are going to have a conversation, make it meaningful. It starts by being purposeful in your speech. If you are going to speak, make it something worth hearing. Ask someone a meaningful question about them, and then listen. I know it sounds crazy, but trust me. Take a moment, and really care. Your world will change. You will become a good listener, and learn to appreciate people more. Others will begin to feel the genuineness behind your questions and attentiveness. You will begin to take notice when there is idle chatter and how it accumulates like static in your mind. After a while you will be able to disengage and avoid it all together. You will truly connect with others and bring more meaning into your relationships at home, work, school, and even with yourself.

3. DEDICATE SOMETHING

Dedicate something, some action or work that you do daily. Attaching work or effort to something truly worthwhile can have a transformative effect on an individual. We see this principle in action all the time with telethons, marathons, and walks. Everybody gets behind a "Big" idea and pulls together to accomplish a goal.

The CrossFit Community is a world-wide sub-culture of fitness fanatics and performance junkies. They have pioneered the WOD, Workout of the Day, structure of workouts that we see gaining popularity today. CrossFit WODs require an extraordinary amount from an individual and are known to leave you lying on the ground gasping at the end, a beautiful site to see depending on which side of the work out you are on. But what makes it work? What drives everyone daily to what many would view as torture?

CrossFitters do a very unique thing; a number of their WODs are named after fallen heroes. Many CrossFit groups are made up of first responders, police, firemen, or military that need a superior level of fitness so that they can be one step ahead of whatever is thrown at them from day to day. They are tightly woven communities in which people form lifelong bonds. When one is lost in the line of duty, their fellow comrades will design a work out in their honor and share it with the larger CrossFit community. It is then posted and efforts are dedicated to the memory of this individual for that day. In this way, they are remembered and memorialized, literally across the globe.

CrossFitters have harnessed their own humanity and compassion to drive their fitness to elite levels. It is genius. It is a living example that when you attach your goals to something bigger than you, something that you can take a part of and have some kind of connection to, it will help you to do more than you ever thought possible before. If you have a huge goal or dream you are trying to achieve, dedicate all of your efforts towards that goal. In this way, you can bring all of your mental and emotional capacity to bear. Dedicate your efforts and watch yourself become more compassionate and successful at your endeavors.

4. STAY POSITIVE

Staying positive is a mental challenge. Remember that negativity can come from all directions, family, friends, colleagues at work, school, and even you. It can be you directing it at others or at yourself. Take a step back and really listen to yourself. Are you abusive in your thought patterns towards yourself? Do you say things to yourself in your head that you would never say to another individual? We aren't perfect, but we are always perfectly positioned for our own growth and personal evolution. Approach yourself with love, and respect your own and others' place on the path. Use affirmations to reinforce your decisions and to maintain your focus.

Affirmations can be words, quotes from great people, inspiring music, imagery that gives you strength, focus, determination, and positive motivation. They can help you at your weakest and when you will be most willing to give up. When challenged, you fill your mind and 'steel your will' with those affirmations and nothing else. As you break down barriers, you will be ready for whatever comes your way.

PERSPECTIVE

All of these exercises are "mental". They help link the physical body with the aspirations of the soul. They are small markers that help lead us to a more fulfilling way of life because they remind us to connect and find purpose.

We must connect, center ourselves, and then direct our intentions. The arrow aims with greater precision not because the point has been sharpened, but because the archer focused his intent. When it comes to finding fitness and wellness with soul, ...let your body be the bow, the mind be the arrow and your soul be the target. This connected meaningful precision will be the map that will guide you along the way.

PULLING IT ALL TOGETHER

The definition of human being is as such: “hu” means halo or light, “man” means mental or mind, and “being” means the present, or the now. This very literal definition of what we are, mental, light beings, living in the now, completely embodies the essence of mind, body and soul (light).

Wellness thrives on this balance. Most of us have the connection with this physical body because it is right before us in plain sight. If it pains, we will feel. If it weeps, we will be showered with tears. If it excites, the heart will race. The body seeks attention from us through proper maintenance and care: physical movement, proper nutrition, and good hygiene.

Similarly with the mind, we hear its constant chatter everyday in every way; even as our bodies rest, this intelligent source dreams and creates new story lines for us. The mind attains balance through positive thoughts and relationships, right speech and daily actions or lifestyle. It finds peace through breath control, meditation and stillness.

The soul in balance, supported by the mind and body, is connected to its source, to its community, to its love. By going within, we tap into this inner oasis where all things are possible. It is the soul that informs the mind, which tells the body. It keeps us aligned and progressing towards that which in essence is our path, our purpose, our manifestation ...of a great life. Whatever it is that makes your heart sing, do it. Leave nothing on the table. Go ahead and march on to greater expansion of your life through a renewed sense of self and spirit. May it be said that when the sun sets on your life, you connected with your Soul and did everything your heart desired. Blessings to you along your path.

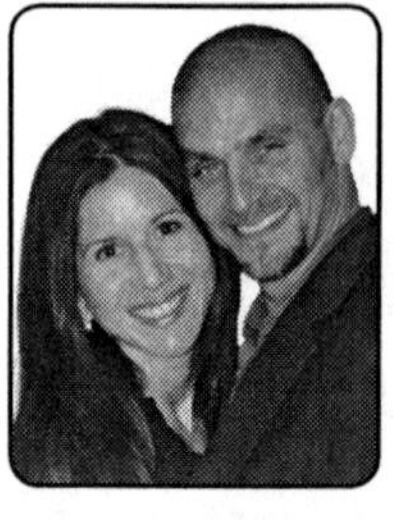

ABOUT THOMAS

Thomas has been teaching martial arts and fitness to all ages for more than 14 years. Spending seven years of that time as a middle school writing teacher, Thomas spent a lot of time studying how the high ideals of his martial arts practice could be used to reach the troubled hearts of his young students. While many of them at the time lived with single parents due to gang violence and crime, Thomas found that by showing them how to expect more from themselves they could tap into the more noble side of their nature.

After teaching, Thomas went on to open his own martial arts and fitness studio where he helps his students see that their true teacher lies within and that they are far more powerful than they realize. Thomas is a 10th generation Sifu, master instructor, of the Northern Shaolin Seven Star Praying Mantis system of Kung Fu. He is also a certified CrossFit trainer, and an RKC, Russian Kettlebell Challenge, certified trainer. He also teaches Qigong, meditation, and loves a cold pint.

ABOUT CLAUDIA

Claudia came to the U.S. with her family fleeing the communist revolution of Nicaragua. From that very instant she was determined to manifest what was being offered by this country. Amnesty was granted to all political refugees and therefore a chance for unlimited potential. She paid her own way through school and graduated from the University of Texas Business School, and then received Culinary training and certification at the Natural Epicurean for Culinary Arts in Austin, TX. Claudia is a Registered Yoga Teacher for both adults and Children. She has been teaching her love of yoga and healthful cooking classes for the past eight years. She has also led several women's retreats on wellness, helping others achieve a greater sense of health in their lives. She is mother to a radiant little girl, Isa, a lover of all animals and a servant to this amazing Earth.

Her passion is for helping others attain wellness and their own truth in happiness.

Thomas and Claudia have known each other since they were in kindergarten and attended grade school through college together. Their connection has always been apparent since they were very young, both attest to having had this soulful bond from the very beginning. It has been their pleasure to share the fruits of their passions, and to help others realize their dreams.

Thomas and Claudia own and teach at their own Health and Family Fitness Facility called Del Sol Martial Arts & Fitness in Austin, TX, they specialize in wellness with Kung Fu, Yoga, CrossFit, Kettlebells, and Healthy Cooking.

STEP 2

NUTRITION

CHAPTER 10

BREAKING THE PLATEAU – IT'S ALL ABOUT THE JOURNAL

BY BRAD & CYNTHIA LINDER

The dreaded plateau. To anyone who has reached a weight loss goal, there is always a point where the progress seems to slow down almost to a screeching halt. The individual continues to follow the steps that got them their initial success, but success is no longer being achieved. The old adage of "calories in – calories out" is what science has explained to be true. When you lose weight you need to eat less in order to continue losing weight. How do you figure out how to eat less without feeling like you are starving yourself? Start keeping a journal and you will break the plateau.

People keep track of many things. At the top of the list are bank statements, kids' schedules, doctors' appointments, grocery lists and needs for the home. People use calendars so they know what they need to do and when they need to do it. But, when it comes to eating, it is typically a mindless and effortless task. The majority of people eat what is convenient, when it is convenient. When someone wants to start making healthier changes, they may put more effort into their eating plans such as getting more fruits and vegetables, eating clean proteins and getting enough water. This is a good first step, but we come across countless individuals that get frustrated with their lack of weight loss results, despite their efforts to exercise and eat right.

Let's look at Ivette, a client of ours that joined our program in April of 2010. She was an ideal client, one who had not exercised in years, needed to lose weight and was committed. She attended class faithfully for the first four weeks and worked hard but had minimal results. Over the next month, Ivette grew in cardiovascular endurance and strength but was not seeing the numbers go down on the scale. Knowing something had to change, she looked to us for advice. We discussed food journaling as well as keeping track of physical activities and abilities. For example, you can write down your meals, but also how many push-ups were done in 1 minute or how long it took to go a half or whole mile. Ivette embraced the idea, committed herself to using this tool, and remained consistent in keeping the documentation. The results were exciting to watch. After the first two weeks, Ivette had lost 2 pounds. The next two weeks, another 2 pounds. For the next 6 months she stayed committed to journaling her foods and exercising and consistently lost 2 pounds every two weeks. That is a solid 25 pounds lost because Ivette simply started to write things down.

When people weigh in and the results they were expecting don't seem to be there, the conversation goes something like this,

"How has your nutrition been?"

"It's good. I don't eat junk like cookies and chips. I eat healthy!"

"Are you writing down what you are eating?"

"Well, I mentally figure that I eat only about 1200-1500 calories a day."

"Do you write it down?"

"No."

"How many cardio workouts have you done this month?"

"Not sure."

This is the number one reason people do not get the weight loss results they were expecting. Guessing and estimating without concretely calculating food and exercise is not going to help you reach your goals. Tracy is another great example. She participated in our 24 Day Challenge and we encouraged her to write down her food and calories. She decided to opt out of keeping a journal because she figured her eating habits were pretty healthy. At the end of the 24 days, Tracy had lost 4 pounds but was disappointed, believing she should have lost more because she was "eating right". Once again we encouraged her to write down her calories just for a week. She agreed after we outlined to her again, that even though she may be consuming good healthy calories, they might still be adding up to a higher total than she thinks. A week later we met with Tracy and she shared with us that since she started journaling, she couldn't believe how many calories she had been consuming even though her food choices were very healthy. After taking a good look at her daily intake, she realized that she was consuming 2000-2500 calories on a pretty regular basis. Despite eating prepared and well-balanced meals and snacks, the calories add up. Healthy choices are encouraged and recommended, but let's look at the calorie intake of unhealthy foods.

In November of 2010, a study was conducted by a nutrition professor from Kansas State University, Mark Haub. Haub wanted to prove that it's not so much the "diet" that you are on, as much as it matters how many calories you are consuming. So, for the next 10 weeks, Professor Haub would consume only 1800 calories. However, those calories would consist primarily of Twinkies, Little Debbie Treats, Doritos and Oreos. He would eat every three hours, eating only up to 1800 calories per day. Included in this total was one protein shake a day, along with a daily multi-vitamin and the occasional can of green beans or a few stalks of celery. By the end of the 10 weeks, he had lost 27 pounds! Although this unbalanced diet is far from recommended, it still proves the point that in order to lose weight you need to consume fewer calories then you are burning on a daily basis.

Another study, published in the *American Journal of Preventive Medicine*, focused on the various weight-loss interventions in more than 1,500 overweight and obese adults. Participants were advised to participate in weekly group sessions, regular exercise, a healthy diet, limited alcohol consumption and the use of a food journal. After five months, participants lost an average of almost 13 pounds, which is a pretty significant amount. However, those who kept up with their food diary more than five days a week lost almost twice as much weight as those who didn't. And perhaps more remarkably, they kept the weight off.

When making the conscious effort to eat healthier, most individuals do make wonderful changes in the fuel they are putting in their bodies. However, too much of a good thing can lead to weight gain. This is where the magic of journaling comes into play. Not only does it keep you accountable, but motivated as well. It creates awareness and responsibility for what is being consumed. When it comes to exercise, writing down your running time can motivate you to go faster the next time you run that same distance. Everyone knows the importance of goal setting, and studies have shown the effectiveness of writing a goal down in order to accomplish it. When someone decides to journal they are far less likely to grab that quick handful of pretzels, eat that harmless piece of birthday cake at the office, finish off the kids leftovers or 'ask for fries with that'. It is this type of mindless munching that can create the surplus, rather then the deficit, which you are looking to create when trying to break that plateau. It's all about the journal.

People are busy. Ask any individual and no one will tell you that they have plenty of time on their hands. Keeping a mental checklist of what you are eating and the exercise you are performing is simply not good enough. Some people can't even remember where they put their keys, so how can they remember accurately not only what they ate, but more importantly, how much they ate. On any given day, a person can rattle off, "Okay, I had a bowl of cereal for breakfast and a cup of coffee, a turkey sandwich and a granola bar for lunch, when I got home from work I had a few cookies, then for dinner I had some spaghetti and meatballs." Seems basic but there are a lot of unanswered questions. What kind of cereal? Did you measure it out to the approximate serving size? What kind of milk was in your cereal? Did you measure that out, too? What kind of bread was your turkey sandwich on? Any cheese with that? What kinds of condiments were used, if any? What did you have to drink with lunch? What type of granola bar was it? What does "a few cookies" mean? Were they large or small? Did they have peanut butter or chocolate chips? Were they homemade or from a package? Was the spaghetti whole wheat? How much was your serving size? Did you add cheese?

What did you drink with this meal? Did you have any additional bread?

You can see by all the questions above that having a mental list of what you are eating is really not good enough if you are trying to break the plateau. Other unanswered questions include if there was any physical activity performed that day. A bike ride? Exercise class? A jog? That is also something that can be documented and journaled. Although it is harder to gauge calories burned while exercising, there are approximations that can be made if you are not wearing a heart-rate monitor or other type of personalized calorie tracker. What is important about writing down your exercise? It provides a timeline of the exercise(s) performed and the length of time it took. This additional data can be used as motivation for future workouts.

Everyone burns a certain amount of calories each day – even while sleeping. For a rough estimate, multiply your weight by ten. That is what you should eat in calories to maintain. To lose weight, multiply your weight number by eight. If an individual weighs 200 pounds, then they need roughly 2000 calories for daily basic function. If that individual would like to lose weight, 1600 calories a day would be the goal. Understand that as you lose weight, the amount of calories you need to consume decreases simply because there is less of you, so your body requires less energy to function.

Journaling is a commitment to your health that will help you break that frustration plateau. The next question is what or how to journal. The following three steps will help guide you. It may take just a week to complete all three steps or it could take a month or longer. The point is to simply begin.

Step One is basically writing down what you eat as the day goes by. Keep a small notebook and write down everything that is consumed – both food and drink. You can also write down the time you eat; this will help with your metabolism and cravings. Ideally you will want to aim for 5-6 smaller meals and snacks spaced 2.5 to 3 hours apart. You can also write about your mood or how you felt, as this may be related to when or what you ate. Try to recognize eating patterns, and make changes that will help you feel better and have more energy. After learning more about your habits and having now acquired the habit of journaling, you can move on.

Step Two introduces the self-education of writing down the calories. This is where the real knowledge lies, because it allows you to start understanding serving sizes and portion control. Eating a turkey sandwich consists of many parts: the bread, amount of meat, condiments and any added vegetables like lettuce and tomato. However, it is not that daunting of a task once you get started, because most people eat a lot of the same things everyday. Once you have the understanding of how many calories are in those portions you are eating, then you only have to worry about looking up the new foods you are adding to your diet.

Now that you have the numbers game down, you can start Step Three. Begin documenting your physical activity and really start to see if that deficit is being created. For example, did you go for a walk or a jog? How long did it take you? Did you attend a personal training or group training session? What was the number of repetitions you were able to perform in a given amount of time? Did you clean the house or garden for an extended period of time? Even just writing down activities, such as gardening or house cleaning, can be valuable information. That way, looking back on your week, you can really take an informed look at how active or sedentary your day is. Writing down your exercise may not seem like much, but it can help motivate you to see what you did and try to improve at your next opportunity.

All of this information about journaling is to help your body break out of the plateau. Keeping a health and fitness journal is a commitment, but it is also an invaluable self-education about how you are treating your body. The journal will let you know if you are providing your body with enough physical activity to keep it fit. It also will allow you to see the kind of fuel that is being used to keep your body at a healthy weight. If you are feeling overwhelmed at the idea of documenting all of this information, you need to first ask yourself if changing the way you look and feel is a priority in your life. If it is not, then the commitment will be lost. However, if it is at the top of your priority list, it will become a precious tool for you to begin making those changes today.

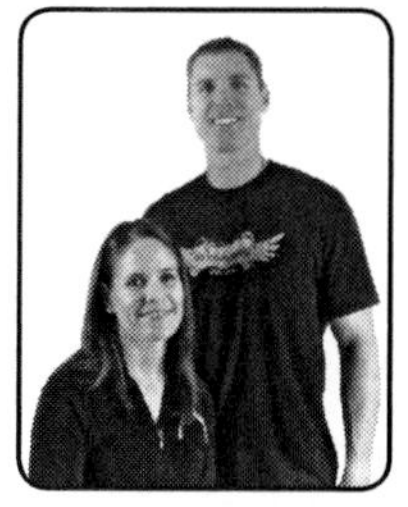

ABOUT BRAD & CYNTHIA

Brad and Cynthia Linder are the owners of Get You In Shape in Coppell, TX.

As a former **professional basketball player, Brad** utilized the knowledge attained from a Master's degree in Health, Kinesiology, and Sport Studies, to optimize his performance. With an extensive background in **fitness** and **nutrition**, he naturally wanted to share this knowledge with others as he entered into the **health** and **fitness** field. Since 1999, Brad has been able to help thousands of participants and clients. Brad has created and produced the Get You In Shape DVD and has been featured as the fitness expert on television and in newspaper articles. Brad has pioneered a high intensity **boot camp** called Get You In Shape Boot Camp, which has received rave reviews. It was featured in The Obama Diaries, by Laura Ingraham.

Cynthia Linder is a former schoolteacher with a Masters Degree in Special Education. She has learned firsthand how to drop dress sizes and get in shape. Struggling for most her adult life to eat healthy and maintain a lifestyle of fitness, she met Brad in 2004. She is now a walking testimony going from a size 10/12 to a size 4/6 and keeping it off. Cynthia has a huge desire to help others by motivating, encouraging, and inspiring others to reach for their goals.

Get You In Shape has grown into one of the leading fitness companies in the Dallas area. What started as one man's mission has grown into a business that offers fitness boot camps, corporate wellness, private training, and nutritional programs. Clients range from high-end millionaires to dedicated housewives. The simple approach of Get You In Shape is to educate, encourage, motivate, and inspire clients to achieve their personal goals. Because of this comprehensive approach to health and wellness, Get You In Shape is ranked in the top tier of fitness businesses in the Dallas, Texas area.

Get You In Shape has a Free Monthly Newsletter list that anyone can subscribe to by going to: www.GetYouInShape.com. You can reach Brad and Cynthia Linder on the web at: www.GetYouInShape.com, by email at: info@GetYouInShape.com or by phone at 214-603-8287.

CHAPTER 11

STAY FULL WHILE INCINERATING FAT ON A REAL FOOD EATING PLAN

BY KEN BOWMAN

Have you tried just about every popular diet out there without lasting success? You may have lost weight on some diets; however in most cases, I bet you couldn't stay on them for an extended period of time. That's because you got tired of being hungry, or you got bored with the limited choices of food, or you were tired from lack of energy.

Eleven years ago I decided to retire from competitive bodybuilding. One of the main reasons for deciding to quit competing was that I was tired of going on restrictive diets to get my body fat to very low levels. I was good at losing fat, but as soon as the show was over I would 'pig out' and gain back most of the fat I had taken off. Sometimes I would end up even more fat than before I started the restrictive diet. Most bodybuilders go through this same process. In fact, almost all dieters go through this process. Chances are that you have too.

When you follow most diets you have to severely restrict or eliminate certain foods or even whole food groups. You may have to severely reduce a macronutrient such as carbohydrate or fat. You end up hungry most of the time and craving foods high in the carbohydrates or fat that you are restricting.

Most of the time since then I was eating the Mediterranean diet. This is a diet of fruits, vegetables, whole grains, legumes, low fat dairy and limited amounts of meat each day. However, I had trouble keeping my body fat from creeping higher while following this diet. Then I read the *Paleo Diet* by Loren Cordain. The Paleo Diet involves eating a diet similar to the diet that human hunters and gatherers ate for about two million years. This is a healthy diet to which our bodies became genetically adapted over time.

With the Paleo Diet, I was able to lose much of the fat that I wanted to lose. But guess what, the same problems arose as before. Even though you're allowed to eat as much meat, fruits and vegetables as you what; you are not to eat any grains, legumes (beans and peanuts), potatoes, dairy and salt. The problem was that I liked bread and grains. I couldn't imagine never eating bread or pasta again. And I like cheese too. Another problem was that I couldn't seem to get full and satisfied with the Paleo Diet. I have since developed a solution to both problems.

THE *'STAY FULL ON REAL FOOD' EATING PLAN*

If you're like most people, you want to eat healthy and lose weight without being hungry or feeling like you want to eat more. You probably don't mind moderating foods, but you don't want to eliminate whole food groups completely.

I have found the perfect way to lose weight while eating all you want of most real foods. This plan has worked for me, my family, and many of my clients. If you what to lose one to two pounds a week and keep it off, keep reading. The *'Stay Full on Real Food' Eating Plan* is a modification of the Paleo Diet. It's sort of like the Paleolithic diet of our ancestors with a sprinkling of the Mediterranean diet. You don't need to totally eliminate any real food from your diet. I'm talking about real food, not junk food and processed food. You will need to drastically reduce processed junk such as refined flour, refined sugar, white rice, fried foods, trans fats, and processed meats. In fact, you should stay away from processed food no matter what diet you are following! Eating this fake food, along with lack of exercise is partly, if not largely, responsible for much of the diabetes, heart disease, cancer, nutritional deficiencies, and obesity in this country.

I have also found two very helpful things to do to help reduce your appetite and give you that full feeling before you even sit down to eat your meal. Drink two full glasses of water 20 minutes before each meal. Before you eat your two heaviest meals you mix a powder in one of the glasses. The powder, called *Calorie Control Weight Management Formula* by Life Extension, has a blueberry-pomegranate flavor and has fat reducing ingredients and a quick gelling fiber that gives you a full feeling and reduces blood sugar levels.

You won't feel hungry on this diet. You can eat all you want of good healthy food. Protein will help satisfy you. Low glycemic carbohydrates (raise blood sugar slowly) will keep your insulin levels from spiking and causing you to overeat. In addition, when you drink two full glasses of water 20 minutes before every meal, you will eat less. Adding the *Calorie Control Weight Management Formula* to one glass of water for your two heaviest meals will make you feel even fuller. Lastly, when you eat a large salad at the beginning of lunch and dinner as recommended, you just don't have much room left in your stomach for large amounts of food.

This is not just a weight loss plan. It is a weight maintenance plan for life. This plan is a very healthy, anti-aging, and performance enhancing plan. You can easily follow this plan for life, because you can eat as much good whole food as you want. Following this diet can significantly lower blood sugar, blood pressure, and blood cholesterol, while giving you more energy and vitality. Don't forget that getting plenty of vigorous exercise is an important component of a healthy lifestyle and will help you burn calories and increase your metabolism.

HERE ARE THE BASIC RULES OF THE 'STAY FULL ON REAL FOOD' EATING PLAN:

1. All the lean meats, fish, and seafood you can eat
2. All the fruits and vegetables you can eat
3. No processed foods

4. Limited amounts of whole grains, beans, potatoes, dairy products, nuts and seeds, dried fruit, and alcohol

5. Eat three meals a day with small snacks between when feeling hungry. Always eat breakfast (If you're not hungry when you wake up, you ate too much or too late the night before.)

6. Drink two full glasses of water 20 minutes before every meal. Mix in the *Calorie Control Weight Management Formula* in one of the glasses of water before your two heaviest meals. Once you reach your weight goal, you can reduce the formula to once a day or discontinue it.

7. Eat a large green salad at the beginning of lunch and dinner

8. Exercise in some form at least 30 minutes a day, six days a week.

HERE'S WHAT MAKES THIS PLAN A HEALTHY EATING PLAN AND AN EFFECTIVE PLAN FOR WEIGHT LOSS:

1. You eat large amounts of fiber from fruits and vegetables, and a little from beans and grains. This adds to a full feeling and promotes regularity. When you add *Calorie Control Weight Management Formula* you get even more filling soluble fiber.

2. You eat enough quality protein from meat. Protein helps you feel satisfied. You won't get hungry if you follow the plan. Plus your body uses three times as much energy to digest and metabolize protein as it does carbohydrate or fat.

3. You eat less high glycemic carbohydrates. High glycemic carbohydrates cause a rapid increase in insulin, which then makes you hungry. Fruits and vegetables generally have a low glycemic index.

4. You eat a diet high in antioxidants, vitamins, minerals, and phytochemicals such as polyphenols.

5. You eat low amounts of these fats - saturated fats, trans fats/hydrogenated fats (eat none), and omega 6 fats (corn oil, soy oil, cottonseed oil, sunflower oil, and safflower oil).

6. You eat moderate amounts of good fats – olive oil, flaxseed

oil, avocado oil, walnut oil, and especially fish oil (fish oil provides DHA & EPA which are very important essential nutrients). If you don't eat oily fish (wild salmon, sardines, mackerel, tuna, anchovies, and others) at least once a week, you should be taking fish oil supplements.

7. You drink plenty of pure water, which not only helps you stay full, but is essential to every process in the body.

8. You get enough exercise, which is a very important component of a healthy lifestyle and will help you incinerate body fat.

When you crave something sweet, have some fruit. Fruit is nature's sweet. Eat some berries for desert or have half of a cantaloupe for a snack. You can also have some dried fruit and nuts, but limit it to a hand full. Your craving for candy and junk food will diminish over time on this eating plan. However, we all have some foods that we will miss. That is why you are allowed one "free meal" a week to eat something not on the eating plan.

The free meal is not a license to 'pig out' on everything you haven't been eating, but a release valve as you get accustomed to the plan. For example, let's say your friends invite you for pizza. Go ahead and have pizza. I would advise you to have a salad first, so you don't eat too much. Or maybe you really miss chocolate. Then go ahead and have a chocolate bar as your free meal. I would recommend that you have it after a full meal, so that you are much less temped to eat more than one.

Eat snacks between meals when you are hungry. Try fresh fruit, raw vegetables, beef jerky, hard-boiled egg (limit 7/week), leftovers, or nuts (limit 4 oz).

When dining out it should not be that hard to eat right. Just remember to drink two glasses of water before you order. Mix the *Calorie Control Weight Management Formula* in one glass if it is appropriate (maybe not at a business lunch or on a first date). Order a salad and the leanest meat available. Better yet, order seafood. Don't forget to get it baked, broiled, grilled, roasted, or sautéed. Try to get some fresh fruit or vegetable at every meal.

EAT ALL YOU WANT OF THESE FOODS

All vegetables (except potatoes, legumes and grains)

All fruit (except dried fruit)

All lean meat

This includes lean beef, lean pork, turkey, chicken, buffalo, wild game, seafood, and eggs (limit to seven a week). Meat should be from grass-fed free range animals when possible. Fish should be wild not farmed, and should be eaten frequently. Meat should be cooked with very little added fat – broiling, baking, roasting, sautéing, or stir frying with a little canola oil, but never deep frying. Always remove skin or cut off fat. If you buy ground beef, turkey or chicken be sure it is lean (90% or more fat free).

Water (add lemon or lime if you want, or use unsweetened seltzer water)

EAT THESE FOODS IN MODERATION

What do I mean by eating these foods in moderation? Limit these foods to no more than one serving a day. You can have a turkey sandwich for lunch. This would be your time to use whole grain bread (preferably the whole grain sandwich rounds that you can find at grocery stores). Another example would be to put low fat cheese in an egg omelet. You can use olive oil & vinegar or a light salad dressing with each of your salads.

<u>Whole</u> grains and breads from <u>whole</u> grains – wheat, barley, rye, buckwheat, millet, quinoa, rice, corn, amaranth, oats

Legumes (beans and peanuts)

Potatoes

Dried fruit – handful (4 oz) as a snack or treat

Low fat dairy products- yogurt, milk, cheese

Nuts and seeds – handful as snack

Oils - use olive oil and flaxseed oil for salad dressing and canola oil for cooking at high temperatures. Use oil sprays with canola oil for cooking in a pan.

Alcohol - wine (one 4-ounce serving), beer (one 12-ounce serving), spirits (4-ounces). You can have two servings of the above on special occasions.

Condiments – limit mayonnaise (light only) to minimum amount to cover whole grain bread or bun, catsup (no more than a tablespoon), soy sauce (one tablespoon or one packet). No need to limit mustard, hot sauce or spices.

AVOID THESE FOODS

Refined flours and foods made from refined flours

White rice

All sugars, candy and sweets (cane sugar, corn syrup, honey, agave, maple syrup, dextrose, and artificial sweeteners – use Stevia or a small amount of honey or agave to sweeten coffee or tea)

All soft drinks

Fruit juices and fruit drinks (they lack the fiber of fresh fruit and have a higher glycemic index)

Fatty meats – bacon, ribs, regular ground beef, lamb

Full fat dairy – milk, cheese, yogurt, ice cream

Deep fried foods

Trans fat (hydrogenated oil) and butter

Most omega 6 oils – corn oil, soybean oil, cottonseed oil, sunflower and safflower oil

The *'Stay Full on Real Food' Eating Plan* is not a quick-fix diet to go on for a few weeks. It is a lifelong healthy-eating plan. If you are overweight and follow this plan, you will gradually lose weight. If you have been eating a lot of poor food choices, you will have a dramatic drop in weight at first. When you normalize your weight, you will be able to maintain your weight permanently. You will be eating delicious healthy food. Real food – not fake food.

For more information, such as adaptations for post workout meals, personal training, boot camp, and to order Calorie Control Weight Management Formula, go to www.KenBowmanBodyCoach.com.

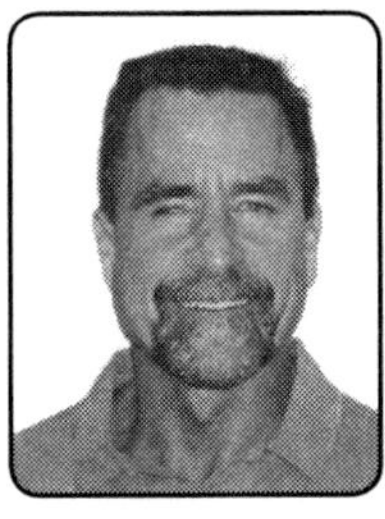

ABOUT KEN

Ken Bowman is passionate about nutrition and fitness. He has been in the health industry most of his life. During college, he worked in a health food store and as a trainer at a health club. He has worked as a trainer in the pharmaceutical industry, where he taught pharmaceutical reps about conditions such as diabetes and hypertension. He has given talks to the public on topics such as 'delaying cognitive decline.' He now owns his own natural food store and is a personal trainer.

As a skinny kid, Ken wanted to put on muscle, so he took up bodybuilding. As a 'hard gainer', he did not get results at first. Then he learned how to train and eat for strength and size, which is now one of his specialty areas as a personal trainer. Ken entered a local bodybuilding contest while in college and won. Since then, Ken has taken first place in several bodybuilding contests, including a comeback contest at the end of 2010.

Ken has been a certified personal trainer for 16 years. He has worked at various training studios and fitness centers as a personal trainer and nutritional consultant. In 2010, he founded Ken Bowman Body Coach. Ken works in Orlando, Florida using the vast knowledge he learned from bodybuilding and years of study to help others reach their fitness goals. In addition to his personal training certifications, Ken is certified as a Sports Nutrition and Body Composition Specialist. Ken specializes in the following areas: 1. Hard gainers, 2. Baby boomers, and 3. People wanting to lose that last 15 pounds or so. Ken also helps men and women prepare for bodybuilding and figure contests.

Ken conducts boot camps and is available for personal training sessions, small group training, and nutrition consultations. For more information regarding his services or pertaining to the *'Stay Full on Real Food' Eating Plan*, such as adaptations for post workout meals, and to order *Calorie Control Weight Management Formula*, go to:

www.KenBowmanBodyCoach.com

CHAPTER 12

"DISCOVER THE OFTEN OVERLOOKED 'SECRET' TO RAMPING UP YOUR METABOLISM, BURNING FAT LIKE CRAZY, AND GETTING MAXIMUM RESULTS IN MINIMUM TIME FROM YOUR HEALTH AND FITNESS PROGRAM"

BY HUT ALLRED

It's no mystery, but the real secret to getting serious results from your program is almost always overlooked and glossed over. Most folks say "I know that already" or "I understand," but in reality they have no clue what they're talking about.

So, what's the secret? -- ***It's your nutrition habits.***

There's nothing more important to your success than building a solid foundation of healthy nutrition and supplementation habits into your life.

Here are the six components of a successful health and fitness program. They include:

1. ***Nutrition*** - the foundation of all health and fitness
2. ***Supplementation*** - to fill in the voids in your nutrition program
3. ***Resistance training*** - to build lean muscle and ramp up the metabolism
4. ***Cardiovascular exercise*** - to optimize fat burning and heart health
5. ***Flexibility*** - to prevent injury and promote recovery from exercise
6. ***Coaching*** - knowledge, support and accountability to get you to the finish line

Right now, I'm going to focus on components 1 and 2, because without that solid foundation, *NOTHING*, and I mean *NOTHING* – ... *WORKS!!!*

It literally makes …

ALL THE DIFFERENCE BETWEEN YOUR SUCCESS OR FAILURE!

But before I get into what to eat and the nutrition habits you MUST instill in your life, let's talk about why nutrition is so important to your results.

First of all, it's essential to increasing your energy. If you're going to increase your exercise activity level, you've got to have the energy to do so. Not only to keep up with all the day-to-day activities you have on your plate right now, but more importantly you've got to have more energy before you even think about adding additional exercise activity into your life!

Second, eating certain foods stimulate the digestive processes of the body in a big way. That's a little known secret to ramping up your metabolism, so I want you to understand what I mean. When you specifically feed your body certain foods, or combination of foods, at periodic intervals throughout the day, you stoke your body's natural metabolic fire (metabolism) and keep it burning hot - kicking your body into fat-burning overdrive.

Third, food is required to provide your body with the necessary nutrients to build and repair muscle. Without the right proteins or amino acids in your body, you simply can't repair tissue, recover from your workout, and gain more muscle. And building more muscle not only allows you to get stronger, but allows your body to *burn more fat all day long.* Ultimately, creating healthy nutrition habits will not just allow you to get and stay fit, but *will improve your long-term health and prevent future disease.*

And that, my friend, is why nutrition is very important.

By focusing on developing solid nutrition habits you not only get results in the short term, but establish the foundation necessary to maintain those results for life!

DO YOU SUFFER FROM ANY OF THESE COMMON SYMPTOMS ASSOCIATED WITH POOR NUTRITION?

There are many symptoms associated with poor nutrition, and you're probably dealing with several of them right now. Any of these sound familiar to you?

- Slow metabolism
- Low energy
- Fatigue
- Slow recovery from exercise
- Excessive soreness after your workouts
- Energy highs and lows
- Poor sleep
- Sugar cravings
- Frequent colds and flu
- Allergies
- High cholesterol
- High blood pressure
- Muscle aches and cramping
- Poor gains in strength
- Poor endurance

If any (or all) of these symptoms ring true don't worry. You're not alone.

Most Americans are suffering from many, if not all, of the above symptoms every single day of their lives. *Why?* Because the Standard American Diet (SAD) is absolutely horrible.

Have you taken notice of all the processed foods and junk you're eating at every turn?

The majority of these symptoms are the direct result of not feeding your body the nutrients required to be fit and healthy. Furthermore, these symptoms indicate much bigger problems are present. What problems you ask?

MORE THAN JUST SOME NAGGING SYMPTOMS, ULTIMATELY BIGGER PROBLEMS ARE CAUSED BY POOR NUTRITION HABITS

Being run down every week, sick several times a year and generally not feeling well is indicative of a much more serious problem with your health - a weakened immune system.

Second, being tired in the afternoons, tired when you wake up, running out of gas at 2:00 pm everyday, and even getting low grade headaches are the direct results of blood sugar fluctuations. When your blood sugar is going up and down throughout the day, insulin levels start fluctuating in the body which takes your body out of the "fat-burning mode"- all of which makes it virtually impossible to lose weight.

Third, being sore for several days after a workout, waking up so stiff you can't move, and only getting slow gains in strength from your exercise program are not normal. These symptoms indicate that RECOVERY from exercise is not being properly addressed. Specifically, I mean taking the right steps nutritionally to stimulate the recovery process after every single workout to get optimum results.

WHAT CAUSES THESE NAGGING SYMPTOMS AND PROBLEMS?

Allow me to dive into a little more explanation. It's important you "get this" today.

1. *Missing meals*. Most clients I work with are eating maybe one or two good meals a day, generally not taking in any healthy snacks in-between, and ultimately eating a big meal every six or seven hours. That doesn't work.

2. *Food processing*. When foods are processed, they lose many of the micro-nutrients (vitamins and minerals), that are naturally present in them. So what happens is we're eating food, but we're not getting the nutrition we need from that food. Unfortunately, unless you're growing your own food on a farm, the majority of food around us today is all processed in some way and void of many nutrients.

3. *Low protein in the diet*. If we don't have enough protein in our diet, then we can't repair tissue or build new lean muscle. In fact, we end up losing what little muscle mass we do have, which you ABSOLUTELY don't want to do. This occurs when there are not enough amino acids present in the bloodstream. The body will then actually break down its own muscle tissue to feed itself- ***essentially eating its own muscle!***

   Most people are not consuming any type of protein at the most important meal of the day- breakfast! You've got to start the day off right to get your body going and that includes eating protein with breakfast.

What "Catabolic" Really Means: When the body is breaking down its own tissue, this is referred to as a *catabolic state*. Ever hear of the character "Hannibal the Cannibal" from the movie Silence of the Lambs? If not, then let me just share with you that this guy was a cannibal - meaning he ATE other people.

When YOU don't eat enough protein, you're body eats itself! I hope that paints enough of a detailed picture for you to understand how bad this really is. You MUST eat enough protein everyday so your body doesn't have to eat itself!

4. *Lack of fiber in the diet.* Another big problem which leads to a whole host of issues, but also impacts blood sugar fluctuations. When this happens your body comes out of the fat burning mode and starts storing fat. This is the exact opposite of what you want to occur.

5. *Ignoring the importance of post-workout nutrition.* Not feeding your body the correct nutrients after the workout leads to slow recovery, slow results, and a lot of unnecessary soreness.

So now that you know the causes of these problems, where do you start to improve?

SIX HIGHLY EFFECTIVE HABITS OF THE HEALTHY, FIT, AND FIRM

There are six healthy nutrition habits that are essential to your progress. *Let's talk about them and why you need to start integrating them into your daily routine right now.*

1. ***Increase your meal frequency***. Strive for five to six "mini-meals" per day. By that, I mean taking the total calories for the day, dividing them by six and having a "mini-meal" every three to four hours. That way you're balancing your caloric intake over the day. This is critical to keeping your metabolism going and really ramping it up. Doing so ensures you're keeping blood sugar levels stable in your body and maintaining a muscle-building, fat-burning state.

2. ***Balance your meals***. We should always have a balance of lean protein sources, low-glycemic carbohydrates, fruits, vegetables, good fats and fiber. Every meal should be balanced with about twice the amount of carbohydrates as protein, and a little bit of healthy fat to provide satiety, so that you're giving your body the essential fats needed to be lean and allow optimal function.

3. ***Drink enough water throughout the day to keep your body hydrated***. Hydration is so important to keeping your body functioning optimally. Water flushes out your kidneys, liver

and keeps everything running clean. If you're not drinking enough water, the kidneys can back up, and then the liver has to help and can't do its job of breaking down fat properly.

You're Not Hungry, You're Dehydrated! A lot of times when people feel hungry, they're not. They're just dehydrated. If you drink enough water, your body will be balanced and function the way that it's meant to. This is very important to aid the release of stored fat.

A good rule of thumb is 8-12 glasses per day. If you live in a warmer, more humid climate or are very heavy right now, then even more is required. In Texas, I generally recommend my clients drink at least from ¾ to 1 full gallon of water per day.

4. ***Take a vitamin/mineral supplement everyday***. All the research today shows that we simply don't get all the nutrients we need in our bodies from our food alone. That's why every major medical and health organization in the country now recommends that everyone take a daily multi-vitamin/ mineral supplement. Notice the word "daily." Not when you remember it, not if you happen to think about it, but every single day. Don't miss. Vitamins and minerals (also called micro-nutrients), are food too, just like carbohydrates, fats and proteins (macro-nutrients) are.

   Just as you can't eat all of your protein for the day in one sitting, nor can you just feed body micronutrients at one sitting or every other day either. Therefore, I recommend you break up your vitamin/mineral supplementation into a serving in the morning with breakfast and again in the evening with dinner. Always take with food for best absorption.

5. ***Use meal replacement shakes and bars for snacks and meals on the go.*** For snacks and convenient meals on the go, good meal replacement products are a must. Remember when I talked about eating 5 to 6 "mini-meals" per day? I don't know anyone who can realistically do that without using a meal replacement product to get through the day. Meal replacement

products include both bars and shakes, but shakes are always going to be a better choice. Generally speaking, they contain less preservatives and unnecessary ingredients. (They don't have to have to be kept in a wrapper on a shelf for a long time like a bar.)

Shake products also generally contain much higher fiber content, without tasting like a brick (like so many bars do). Plus they're simple and convenient to prepare. All you have to do is mix it up in milk or water. Use them for in-between meals and those days when you don't have time for a full breakfast or need a healthy meal on the go.

Road Warrior Tip: When traveling, eating right is very challenging. Often ordering a healthy meal for lunch or dinner in a restaurant is not so bad, but finding a good breakfast and getting in healthy snacks is a challenge. This is a great time to pack extra meal replacement bars and shakes with you to keep you on track with your nutrition program.

6. ***Always take a recovery shake after your workout.*** Get into the habit right now. It will pay dividends later. Post workout nutrition dramatically speeds up the recovery process. It will reduce your soreness, maximize your release of anabolic hormones (like growth hormone and testosterone), and allow your body to maximize building muscle and burning fat.

   When you consume a well-balanced shake after exercise, carbohydrate stimulates insulin to drive the branch between amino acids (protein) to the muscle cell. That way you can maximize recovery and get right back in the gym again very soon – ensuring faster results from your program.

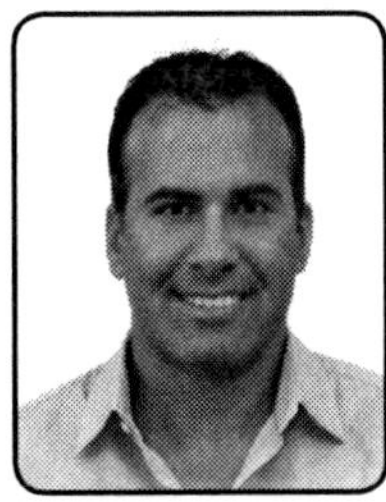

ABOUT HUT

A native of Brownwood, TX, Hut Allred's journey into the world of health and fitness began as a standout athlete in all sports, especially football. He was team captain, named to multiple all-state teams, and earned an athletic scholarship to the University of North Texas.

While at the University of North Texas, Hut was able to continue his success on the playing field. He was a four-year letterman, team captain, all-conference selection, and was a Doak Walker nominee as one of the top Division 1A running backs in all of collegiate football.

Not long after graduating from the University of North Texas, Hut decided to jump head-first into building a career in the fitness industry. In 2000, Hut became certified as a personal trainer by the American Council on Exercise (ACE) and began training and coaching individuals on the benefits of exercise and a healthy lifestyle.

Hut's next project involved founding a personal training company in 2002, aptly named New Wave Fitness, Inc., which quickly grew to include a staff of 10 trainers and providing services throughout the Dallas / Fort Worth area. Hut has personally coached hundreds of clients to reach their health and fitness goals.

Coaching and educating eventually led to writing. Hut has authored a fitness book for the Fit Corp USA company entitled ***"How To Get Maximum Results In Minimum Time From Your New Home Fitness Equipment"*** which is used to help customers of Fit Corp USA get the best results from their fitness products.

With his fitness expertise, as well as warm, friendly, and approachable character, Hut has become a captivating and much sought after speaker on the topics of nutrition and health. He has contributed articles regularly to E-fitness and other health related sites; his health and fitness writings have also found homes in two national magazines and several local publications.

Hut is now focused on expanding his company and currently does a tremendous amount of speaking, writing, and consulting.

To learn more about Hut Allred, and how you can receive free special reports and other invaluable fitness information from one of the country's leading experts, visit: www.NewWaveFitness.com or call Toll-Free 1-866-230-5460.

CHAPTER 13

NUTRITION TO 'KICK START' YOUR METABOLISM

BY RANDY HARTZ

The hardest part about losing weight is gaining momentum. It seems like every person I talk to, who wants to make a physical change, struggles with getting started. We all talk about speeding up our metabolism but no one really gives us any concrete method on how to do it.

Your metabolism is simply the rate at which your body burns through calories. Some of us have fast metabolisms but unfortunately many are very slow. Typically, those with slow metabolisms blame it on genetics – implying that it is completely out of their control. They believe they are simply cursed with a slow metabolism with no hope of changing it.

Genetics do play a part but the truth is you have created your metabolism as a result of your eating and exercise habits. It's difficult to take a look in the mirror and say I have no one to blame but myself for where I am. Until you are willing to do that, all the nutrition tips and tricks in the world aren't going to help. The good news is that from this point on you can recreate your eating habits and speed up your metabolism as a result. This will be the catalyst in helping you reach your goals.

Every person that I meet with wants to make some kind of a physical change. It may be weight loss, toning up, or just looking good in a swimsuit. The first step is to get you feeling better. That leads to the next step which is increasing your performance. That may be getting off the couch and going for a walk or to the gym. The result of these two steps is looking better. Unfortunately we often try to skip the first two steps and jump right to looking better. Hey, we live in a 'quick-fix' society and the only thing better than having it right now would be having it yesterday, right?

I have a simple plan to help you implement this process of feeling better to increase your performance, which will end up leading you to your goal of looking better naked. That's really what we are trying to do here. Feeling better about how we look increases our confidence and spills out into every other area of our lives. Let's face it, if you are feeling good and full of energy, everything else in life tends to go better.

I learned an interesting thing recently. With all of the garbage we typically put into our bodies, we are not assimilating the nutrients we are putting in. Simply put, I could write you the most complete diet plan in the world, but if your body is not digesting and absorbing those calories it is worthless. There are a few reasons for this.

Artificial sweeteners are the first culprit. Did you know it takes roughly 15 weeks for one packet of artificial sweetener to go through your body? Many people think drinking diet soda is ok because there are no calories in it. The problem is these artificial sweeteners begin to coat the lining of the digestive system making it difficult for the good nutrients to pass through and get into the blood stream. The average American has about 3½ pounds of artificial sweeteners stuck in their digestive tract at any one time.

Preservatives are another problem that affect proper digestion. Just because you eat something that has a preservative in it doesn't mean that the preservative quits preserving. They act like toxins in your body and are hard to get rid of in certain organs such as the colon and the liver. Over the long term, they hurt digestion and cause all kinds of negative side effects. I know it is next to impossible to cut out all preservatives, but I have some solutions that will help you out.

The last problem that affects your body's ability to absorb nutrients is antibiotics. They are great at killing the bad bacteria that is in your body that causes you to be sick. Unfortunately they can't differentiate between bad and good bacteria and they end up killing it all. My four-year old just got done with a round of amoxicillin for a bacterial infection. Now he is struggling with constipation because the healthy bacteria are not in his lower intestine to break down the foods correctly and aid in digestion. This healthy bacteria needs to be replaced after a round of antibiotics to restore proper intestinal health.

The question you should be asking yourself right now is what does this have to do with kick-starting my metabolism? Glad you asked. If artificial sweeteners, preservatives and antibiotics are not allowing your digestive tract to be as efficient as it needs to be then you have a major problem. The average 38 year old female actually only absorbs about 22% of the calories she consumes compared to the average 18 year old that absorbs roughly 90%. Remember when you could eat pizza and ice cream and it wouldn't affect you and now if you even look at it you gain 5 pounds? Proper digestion is a major factor.

The majority of people that I coach have the belief that to lose weight they have to eat less. If you buy into this mentality when you are ready to lose weight you will cut your intake of calories down. Your body only recognizes the calories that are absorbed and make it to your cells not the calories that you consume. If you were consuming 2000 calories per day and you only absorbed the average 22% that would mean your body was only recognizing 440 calories per day. You go on a diet and cut your intake down to 1400 calories per day so that 22% turns into just over 300 calories per day. Again, your metabolism only recognizes the calories that make it to the cells not the calories you eat. Talk about starvation!

The solution is to prepare your body to absorb the nutrients that we put in. Here are seven keys to helping you kisckstart your metabolism through proper nutrition.

The first key is going through a cleanse program. We want to strip all the artificial sweeteners, preservatives and restore the healthy bacteria in our gut. The one I recommend is a ten day product sold through a nutritional company called Advocare. There are a ton of cleanse products on the market but with everything there is good and bad. The right cleanse should have probiotics to replace the healthy bacteria that your body needs. It should also contain a high quality fiber to help clean out the insides and restore healthy digestion. You should not have to go on a crazy nutrition plan during the cleanse phase like a liquid only diet.

Initially, you may think cleansing is going to have some nasty side effects and keep you in the bathroom all day. This cleanse is gentle and doesn't send you running to the bathroom – it just makes that time more productive. You will feel lighter, the clothes will fit looser and you will have a better sense of well-being when you are done. My wife was catching the "24 hour flu" on a regular basis. Typically, it is bad bacteria that your body is trying to fight off. Doing a cleanse and adding the healthy bacteria back into her system has made an incredible difference in her health.

The second key I need you to focus on is drinking plenty of water. Over 90% of Americans walk around in a dehydrated state. Drink at least your bodyweight in ounces per day. For ten days cut out the coffee, diet and regular pop, and anything else that is not sugar-free. I add an energy drink packed full of B-Vitamins to curb the caffeine withdrawals and get you feeling great from day one. The product is called Spark and is also from Advocare. It will help to curb cravings and get you feeling better, so you can start performing better which ultimately will lead you to your goals.

The first ten days are used to gain some much needed momentum. I typically try to get my clients quick results to build confidence that the program works and to get them excited to keep pushing forward. Once you start to see progress it gets easier to eat the right nutrients and get your workouts in. Most have tried everything and are so skeptical that this helps them believe that change is possible.

The goal is to have you full of energy and have your appetite under control. A typical diet has you starving, running on willpower, feeling miserable and thinking about food constantly. This is not the environment we are trying to create to burn fat and maintain lean muscle.

Breakfast is the third key on the list to 'kick start' your metabolism. What you eat within the first 30 minutes of the day sets the stage for how your body will perform. A bowl of cereal filled with sugar is not going 'to cut it'. It may be low in fat but there is no protein to support lean muscle and the quality is below average at best. Choose a balanced breakfast that has at least 20 grams of protein and a good quality carbohydrate source like oatmeal or a low sugar cereal. If you absolutely don't have time for breakfast, make a meal replacement shake. The one we recommend contains predigested protein so it gets where it needs to go rather than passing right through your body. You get what you pay for and you don't get what you don't pay for.

The fourth key to success is eating more small frequent meals throughout the day. I know you have heard it before but here is the reason why. If we can control your insulin levels and keep them stable throughout the day, it creates the environment where fat can be burned as fuel. Your metabolism is like a fire. If we can keep that fire burning hot all day long you will simply burn more calories leading you to your goal. This is another reason why traditional diets that have you eating less set you up for failure. Five to six small meals spread throughout the day will guarantee success.

The fifth key is to add a high quality protein in at every meal and snack. How much you need depends on bodyweight and what you are trying to accomplish. Start out with a minimum of 20 grams every time you eat and adjust from there. Women need to focus on this because they tend to skip this step. Protein supports the lean muscle that you have. Don't worry, you aren't going to bulk up, the hormones are not there to support that.

The sixth key is to limit starches three to four hours before you go to bed. It is a myth that you should not eat anything after six o'clock at night. Your body repairs and recovers during sleep and it needs the proper nutrients to do that. The key is choosing lean protein sources instead of a bowl of cereal. A great choice is low-fat cottage cheese.

The seventh and final key is keeping a food journal. *This is so important it should be first on the list.* There is something about having to write down the three cookies you snuck from the lounge at work. Even if no one reads the journal it does an amazing job of holding you accountable. This simple step will multiply your chances of being successful.

To simplify all of this, I use a nutrition plan called the 24 Day Challenge. The average person drops 10 pounds and 10 inches during the program, but the best part is the energy and how great you are going to feel. It takes 21 days to form a new habit or break an old habit. Everything I have shared with you here is simply about new habits. At first it requires discipline, effort and knowing what the end result is going to look like. If you implement these seven keys you will achieve success in your health and fitness.

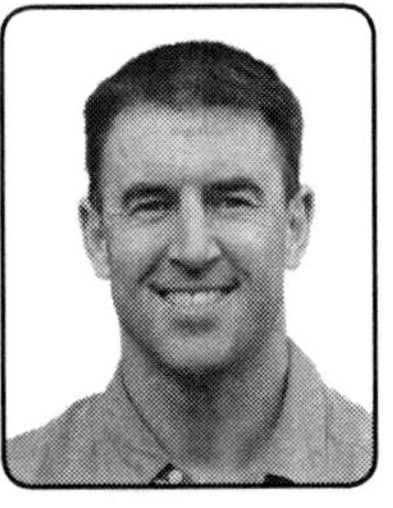

ABOUT RANDY

Randy Hartz is a passionate entrepreneur, speaker and fat loss expert. Since 1995 he has been involved in virtually every aspect of the fitness and weight loss industry – as a gym owner, personal trainer, nutrition consultant and freelance writer.

Randy is a certified personal trainer and a graduate of South Dakota State University holding a degree in Exercise Science. Randy was a competitive bodybuilder for over 10 years and won a national championship in 2001. He was featured in *Muscle & Fitness* and *Flex Magazine*.

Randy is an expert on how the body performs with exercise and nutrition, and uses that information to help people get that lean, toned body that they want, so they can live the quality of life that they deserve. He works day-in and day-out with professionals, corporations and organizations teaching them how to incorporate fitness into their busy lifestyles while focusing on truth and exposing fitness myths.

He spends his free time with his wife and 3 sons. Randy is very active in his local church and enjoys speaking to young people about life lessons and educates them on making the right choices.

RandyHartz@TryonGym.com
605-271-9600
www.TryonGym.com
www.Advocare.com/05082405
www.SiouxFallsBootCamp.com

CHAPTER 14

WHAT KIND OF AN EATER ARE YOU?

BY AUDRA BAKER

Nutrition is a funny thing. If we're not obsessed with the latest diet book, we're going crazy over the next "belly detox". If it's not one program, plan, or quick-fix, it's another, …the never-ending cycle of a multi-billion dollar industry that propels us from one plan to another.

I guess what makes me crazy about the whole thing is that besides the fact that it's confusing for just about anyone, it also makes no sense to tell someone who is smack-down right in the middle of an emotional eating binge to go on a "diet plan," …or telling a fast-food addict to eat grass-fed beef and go shopping at the farmers market.

And I should know. Growing up a "fast food junkie", the only veggies I ate were corn and potatoes (which is really funny, considering corn isn't even a veggie!). Occasionally I was force-fed green beans, but that's about as good as it got.

Growing up in the fat-free 80's and 90's, and falling victim to an overly-sugared and under-nourished diet, brought pure confusion. I struggled with my weight and sugar cravings from a young age, and after sheer frustration, I finally decided 'to take the bull by the horns' by doing tons of research and becoming a Certified Nutrition Educator.

Through this process, I've discovered what truly constitutes a healthy diet and have since healed my body through nutrition. But after figuring it out for myself, and then consulting hundreds of people along their nutritional journey to better health, it's become clear to me that there are very distinct categories of "eaters". It's not a judgment of good or bad, right or wrong, but rather it's an understanding of where you are right now, and it might lead you to some insights about why some programs, diets, or concepts may or may not work for you.

Before you take on any new plan, book, program, nutritionist, etc., take the time to figure out where you lie on this nutritional spectrum. Because how and what you eat truly determines your health and wellness.

LEVEL 5: THE BLISSFUL EATER
LEVEL 4: THE COMPETITIVE EATER
LEVEL 3: THE CONSCIOUS EATER
LEVEL 2: THE BREAKTHROUGH EATER
LEVEL 1: THE EMOTIONAL EATER

LEVEL 1
THE EMOTIONAL EATER

Now before I dig too deep into this topic… who here *doesn't* emotionally eat? If you just said you don't, you're a liar! What holiday can you think of that's not surrounded by food? When's the last time you went to a wedding or a birthday that didn't have cake? Eating is so embedded into our emotions, cultures, and traditions that there's really no way around it. But I really think this is part of the wonderment of being human and connecting with others. And this isn't really the kind of emotional eating I'm talking about. When your eating habits are completely controlled by emotional triggers, the last thing you are really caring about is whether or not something is "good for you." When a food craving hits, which can be caused both by psychological or physiological reasons (usually it's a mix of both), nothing else matters but getting that food into your mouth.

The one crucial step that every single "program" seems to skip over is the insanely complex and intricate webbing of emotions tied into how and why we eat.

Because if it was just as simple as "eat less", and I could give you the exact list of what to eat and you followed it 'to the tee,' there would be no problems and we would all live happily ever after, wearing our bikinis and Speedos on the beach without a care in the world.

But it's not that easy.

Emotions play a huge part in our successes and failures when it comes to choosing the right foods and to weight loss in general. The best diet plans in the world will do you absolutely no good if you're unwilling to stop eating Ben & Jerry's after a long and stressful day at work. No weight loss guru can help you if you can't stop yourself from "trolling" the kitchen unconsciously before and/or after dinner (...or in the middle of the night for that matter).

The underlying issue here is getting your emotional state-of-being in check, so that you will have a greater chance of success at this game.

Now, when we are talking about emotional or compulsive eating (same thing by the way), lets be real here: I'm not talking about labeling emotional eating as "good" or "bad". I'm talking about paying attention as to who is ruling your world: "you" (your higher self) or "your emotions" (your not-so-higher-self).

I was recently listening to a great speaker talk about this exact concept. He was speaking about when people lose all control and blame it all on their emotions. "I just couldn't control myself," he joked. His tone was light and it was quite funny because when it's all said and done, the truth of the matter is that we — our higher selves — are completely in charge of our emotions. There is an internal choice to make. ***We get to decide when we act out emotionally***. If you are used to letting your emotions guide you through life, this may seem unrealistic. But if you listen very closely inside of yourself, there is a moment before the emotion takes over where your 'higher self' has the opportunity to choose one path or the other. It really is within your control.

What I offer my clients are resources and tools to help them overcome this battle.

1. When it comes to emotional eating, the first step is to realize and bring it to your conscious (aka: AWAKE!) mind that you are choosing your food for reasons other than health and life.

2. It's not about judging the above decision, but it's about noticing if it serves you. It might serve you to eat cake at a celebration, or indulge in wine and chocolate on Valentines Day. The question is: 'Does this food I'm about to devour serve me and the higher good of what I want for my life?'

3. If the answer the above question is an unequivocal "no", then it's probably time to take a look at what's going on deeper inside of you. Because if you are emotionally eating and it serves no helpful purpose, then what you are really doing is attempting to solve an emotional problem by putting food in your mouth.

   And here's a little hint that's 100% accurate:- **IT NEVER WORKS! ...Ever!**

   There is no type or amount of food that can fix whatever it is. *Never. Ever. Never.* (Did I get my point across?)

Recently, one of my clients, whom my heart goes out to, just lost her sister. Just hearing her say those words brought tears to my eyes and even as I write this, my heart goes out to her and her family. She was so set with her plans of showing up to her training sessions and eating clean because she's already done the internal work and realized that this is her year to get her health and weight under control (this is indicative of a Level 2 eater we'll talk about next). And as soon as she discovered her sister's untimely death, it all went out the window.

I offer this example to you as a real-life and very valid reason as to why someone would "fall away" from their worthy goals. But tell me, how does food fix anything? It might comfort you in the moment, but then within seconds the pain is still there and now you're 'pissed' because not only is your sister still gone, but also, now you just ate too much 'crap' and feel worse than when you started. The food was an attempt to make the pain go away, but all it did was create more pain. Food will never fix the problem.

What is really needed in this moment is to FEEL THE PAIN. To be so present in the moment that, instead of trying to push the feelings away or stuff the feelings deep down inside, you choose to go a different route, ...you CHOOSE to feel it.

Now, lets get clear here. I'm no therapist. I've have my fair share of "life and wellness coaching certifications" and read enough books and research to understand all of this cognitively, but actually DOING the work (i.e., ...putting the cookie down and choosing to "feel the pain"), is ***really freaking hard.***

But really, it's the only answer to a better, healthier, and more productive life.

And the truth is that you will never completely attain your weight loss and health goals until you can work through your pain and get to the bottom of it. If you find yourself spending most of your time as a level 1 emotional eater, I encourage you to *stop trying out the lastest "diet".... None of them will work.* Instead, start to dig deeper and find out what's really going on. It will change your life for good!

LEVEL 2
THE BREAKTHROUGH EATER

The Breakthrough Eater is on a path to do exactly what it sounds like: literally breaking through all the emotional triggers and bad habits to gain control over their health and eating.

The breakthrough eater is sick of being sick and overweight. They are sick of the cycle of not taking care of their health, overeating on a regular basis, and having their emotions lead their diet and life. This person is actively seeking an answer and will stop at nothing to find it. Often times, something created a "breakthrough moment". Maybe it was a doctor's visit that told them they're a Type 2 diabetic. Or a family member that's very sick triggers the awakening of making their health first priority. Whatever it might be, these are people who are looking for a change and are ready for it.

It's like they've woken up from a sugar-induced coma and are actively seeking answers. This is usually the type of person that will seek out my services. Unfortunately, this is also the type of person who falls victim to a multi-billion dollar diet and weight-loss industry. Bottom line? There's 'a whole lotta crap out there' coated with slick and shiny marketing that would make anyone want to buy in to their empty promises, and because of this, I see many Level 2 eaters gets stuck. They have all the intentions to do the research, to do the work and to find the help, only to fall victim to some random "diet plan" that restricts calories or teaches them to go on a "cookie diet". So after obvious disappointment, the Level 2 Breakthrough Eaters end up right back at a Level 1 emotional state.

Some people spend years, or even their entire lives, reliving this yo-yo effect over and over again.

It is my job, my duty, my calling (whatever you want to call it!) to take a Level 2 eater through the entire process of breaking through this vicious cycle to move into a Level 3 Conscious Eater. It doesn't have to be a painful or challenging process when you have the right coaching, education, accountability, skill set, and mind set. If one of my clients truly comes to me as a Level 2 Breakthrough Eater ready to change their life and get out of the cycle of dieting, I can help. In fact, I've helped hundreds of my clients do just that.

The reason why my clients have such amazing success with this is partly because of the sound, science-based, non-diet approach I offer, but also because there is magic in working with a coach. The encouragement and accountability from not only a professional, but also from someone who's been there before, is often the key to success.

If you find that you are a Level 2 Breakthrough Eater, don't just sign up for the latest infomercial! Do the research to find real answers and credentialed professionals who can help you along your journey. The only path to true long-term success (read: no more yo-yoing!) is through a consistent exercise plan *and* a nutrition plan that teaches you and holds you accountable to lifestyle and eating habits over time. If it sounds like a scam, …it probably is. Nip this in the bud and don't stop until the job is done. By going through the process and committing to finish it to the end, you will never have to 'yo-yo' again. A new healthier life is waiting right around the corner for you!

LEVEL 3
THE CONSCIOUS EATER

This I believe should be a worthy goal for all who have struggled with their weight, food, emotional eating, or just being a part of a diet-crazed society. The Level 3 Eater has a conscious and respectful relationship with food and themselves, and has finally broken free from the death-grip of "dieting".

Becoming a conscious eater is my ultimate goal for my clients and for you. Does that mean that you never ever eat cake again? No, but you do it in a very healthful and respectful way to your body, and it's a very clear and decisive choice. It's a different story having a piece of cake or a bite of something at a birthday versus having a binge at Starbucks. Having a healthy and energetic body that is neither over- nor under-weight, but rather functions at high levels is something that everyone deserves. The only we way we experience this world is through our body and senses. If you spend your whole life in a bio-chemical funk because your hormones are so out of whack from all the processed food and sugar, then surely you are not experiencing all the world has to offer.

The Conscious Eater focuses on foods that are life-giving, minimally processed, and nourishing because instead of being so wrapped up in the diet and weight-loss craze, they are more wrapped up in keeping their body performing at top levels, whether that's making it through a busy day in corporate America or busting out the latest CrossFit work-out. They eat when they're hungry and stop when they're full, instead of binging unconsciously and overeating, all of which are skills learned and implemented while moving through Level 2. The Level 3 eater has mastered this lifestyle shift. And while life will always provide challenges, the Level 3 Conscious Eater has the skill-set and know-how to maneuver through their life without reverting back to using food as crutch.

LEVEL 4
THE COMPETITOR

The Competitor takes their eating to a whole different level of learning how to manipulate their body and performance through nutrition. I love working with Level 4 eaters because they have moved through the struggles of weight loss, learned to become conscious of their choices to live the fullest life possible, and are now seeing the possibility of turning their body into a well-fed machine who can out run, out lift, and out perform their competitors! Professional athletes obviously fall into this category, but there are many people in the general population who are discovering that they too can have excellent levels of fitness, and compete and perform at high levels once they realize the foods they eat completely facilitate this process. And since sports nutrition is a passion of mine, it's a pleasure working with this focused and elite group.

LEVEL 5
THE BLISSFUL EATER: EATING FOR A BIGGER CAUSE

Have you heard of a CSA box? Did you hit the farmers market last weekend? Do you know the name of the ranch where your beef was raised, or even better yet… do you know the ranchers name? Do you grow your own veggies, raise your own hens, or milk your own cow? Okay, maybe I was going a little over top at the end, but then again… you'd be surprised. If you do any of the above, then I might call you a blissful eater. You smell something rotten going on in the food industry and agri-business.

There's a mini-food revolution going on, and many people are taking their health into their own hands and choosing a better way to eat. They are saying goodbye to global food, and choosing to shop locally, organically, and purchasing products that are brought to the market responsibly and ethically. Now, a blissful eater isn't really a level at all as this person very easily can be intermeshed into each of the above types of eaters.

I know plenty of Level 1 Emotional Eaters who shop at the farmers market for their veggies, and also have major sugar addictions, and Level 2 Breakthrough Eaters, learning how to live a healthier life by cleaning up their diet while simultaneously choosing to eat grass-fed beef.

This interesting world of healthy eating and nutrition can be a lot less confusing and even a fun adventure, if you know where you stand. Understanding what level you are at now will give you the necessary road map to make smarter choices, and get a clear picture on where you want to go, as well as if certain plans, programs, or coaches are right for your path.

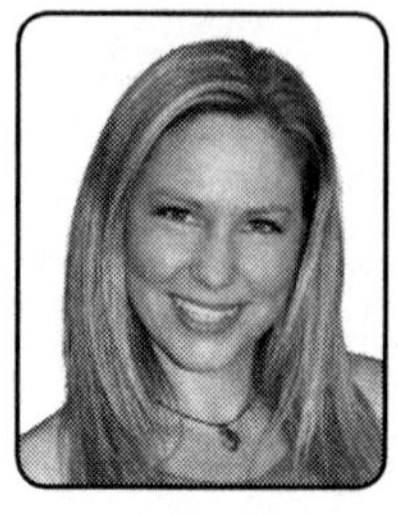

ABOUT AUDRA

With over 15 years experience in the health and fitness industry, Audra owns and operates Be Fit Boot Camps in San Jose, CA, a cutting-edge outdoor fitness program that focuses on group and personal training, and covers the gamut of all elements necessary for success: from motivation and adherence to nutrition, weight loss, and metabolic conditioning. Audra holds a degree in kinesiology and multiple certifications including from the National Academy of Sports Medicine.

After spending enough time frustrated with confusing nutrition misinformation, and dealing with her own struggles of being an overfed, undernourished fast-food junkie, Audra has come a long way. A life-long student of nutrition, she has taken multiple graduate courses in Holistic Nutrition and is a Certified Nutrition Educator and Wellness Coach.

Known as an expert in weight-loss resistance, Audra inspires her clients through her own story of struggle and has developed extensive weight loss and nutrition programs that have helped hundreds of her clients get back on track – living the life they deserve.

Self-proclaimed nerd now trapped in an athlete's body, Audra never played sports as a kid, and spent most of her childhood in a sugar-induced Twinkie-coma. It was from this space where she made the conscious decision to change her life. Now an avid Mountain Biker, Snow Boarder, Surfer, and Salsa Dancer, she has built her career teaching her clients that it's never too late to take control of their health, body, and life.

To learn more about Audra and how you can receive free special reports outlining what it really takes to finally break free from the mental tyranny of losing weight and weight-loss plateaus, visit www.AudraBaker.com or call toll free 1-877-922-3348.

STEP 3

FITNESS

CHAPTER 15

PRENATAL AND POSTNATAL EXERCISE

BY ARIN RALSTIN AND TONY LINDAUER

Over the last few years, we have consistently seen women in their late 30, 40s, and 50s who have high blood pressure, no energy, bad posture, high body fat percentage, little muscle tone, and low self-esteem. When these women decided to seek us out to make life changes, many of the stories we would hear from them were very similar. They would tell us they stopped working out and/or did not work out during their pregnancy. One lady said, "Oh, I just never lost my baby weight and each year went by and I just kept gaining weight." When I asked how old her *baby* was, she said, "15!"

When we would examine these women, we identified a life-changing need to develop pre- and post-natal exercise programs. These women, who were in their 30s to 50s, had lost their self-esteem and let their bodies go because of pregnancy. They should not have to suffer because they wanted to be a mother. From this, we created programs to help women – no matter what stage they are in. It has become a growing trend to see women seeking out a Fitness Professional before they become pregnant, and in several cases they need to get to a healthy weight per their doctor before they could even conceive. It is perfectly safe to start an exercise program while you are pregnant, even if you have never exercised before! You have to search for a qualified Fitness Professional, and work closely with your doctor. The point is, no matter what, being in good overall health is the goal.

Creating pre- and post-natal programs has been life-changing for the new moms and the fitness professional. Each expecting mother gains the confidence, strength, endurance, and will power to know that her body can and will drop the post-baby weight. It is a very gratifying feeling to know you are helping someone with one of the most monumental times of their life!

Not every pregnancy is planned, but rest assured, once you receive the news that you are pregnant it is time to take action. In a perfect world, everyone would plan everything in their life, especially something this important, but this is not reality. The reality is once you are pregnant, things will have to change. We know many of you are thinking, "I have a great plan of action! We have saved plenty of money for medical expenses, time off work, new crib, diapers, new paint for the nursery, and many other essentials for the new arrival." This is very good planning, but what we want to discuss is overlooked in many cases and this is one of the most important factors when one starts to think about pregnancy, ...your health.

Your health and lifestyle can be the main factor in your baby's development. Developing a good fitness plan will improve your chances of having a healthy baby and a safe pregnancy. We recommend starting an exercise program 6 months prior to the process of conception. Please do not worry if you are reading this and are already expecting; it is never too late! The 6 months of planning is geared toward action steps for a healthier lifestyle. Many athletes spend countless hours developing their bodies with exercise and nutrition in preparation for a major event such as a marathon. These athletes understand the benefits and needs of a healthy body and they know with a good workout program and healthy eating, their body will be ready for a major competition. Pregnancy is very much like a major competition when considering the physical and emotional demands that will be presented to your body.

One of the most important items to remember is to start slow. We find several people want to be exactly how they were in high school and they start too fast, too much, and are so sore they quit before they have even started. Just as the amazing Dan John said, "Slow and steady over the long haul." Keep this phrase in mind at all times. Build the body up slowly and increase appropriately over a specific duration of time.

Next, we recommend working with your doctor and seeking out a Fitness Professional. With both of these tools in place you will ensure your safety and well being. Find a Fitness Professional that has great credentials; make sure he or she holds a four year degree in a related field of Exercise Science and a certification with a national organization. Once you have found your Fitness Professional, sit down and identify your goals in writing. Pin point exactly what you want to achieve with your investment in both, and set a schedule that works for you.

In the design of your program to a new and healthy lifestyle, you are going to notice changes in how you feel initially, and then, depending on where you are starting, results are just around the corner. When it comes to exercise, remember that it takes everything working together. Just because you are working out 5 days a week doing various activities does not mean you can just forget about your nutrition. Your nutrition becomes extremely important. With this new plan, incorporate 2 – 3 days of resistance training, 2 - 3 days of cardiovascular training, and a healthy well-balanced meal plan. Stay away from any diets. If you cannot do the diet for the rest of your life, then you should not do it in the first place. We at Transformation Fitness and Wellness recommend 6 small meals per day and to keep your food as natural as possible. Stay away from as many processed foods as possible. If the food can sit on the shelf for multiple months, try to find a fresher alternative. Keep everything in moderation. It is easy to get excited about your new lifestyle, but remember to start slow and be balanced.

During your pregnancy, each week is going to change and it will become essential to check with your doctor along the way to make sure the fetus is developing properly. There are many informative articles on how exercise helps you have a healthy and successful pregnancy. Some key points to keep in mind while exercising are wear a heart rate monitor and keep your heart rate below 140-150 bpm (discuss specifics with your doctor), do not lay on your back after 16 weeks, drink plenty of water all day, monitor how you are feeling, and take breaks often. Watch for any signs and symptoms such as: dizziness, headaches, shortness of breath, chest pain, abdominal pain, and vaginal bleeding. If you experience any of these signs and symptoms, discontinue the activity and consult your doctor. Also do be aware that your core temperature will increase faster while pregnant. Avoid working out in extreme heat, make sure you can carry a conversation, and once again, stay hydrated.

We have had several women deliver their baby, and the doctor goes on and on about how physically fit the mother is. If you are delivering vaginally, having the endurance and strength to push your baby is imperative. Afterwards, your recovery will hopefully be very appropriate and have you back in a few weeks. After you deliver, your doctor will advise you as to when it will be appropriate for you to return to exercise. For a vaginal delivery, six weeks is the recommended time frame to wait. With a cesarean delivery, eight weeks is recommended. We at Transformation Fitness and Wellness always wait for the doctor's clearance before starting an exercise program after the baby is born.

After your baby is born, your world is forever changed! Now there is someone else who is more important and who needs your constant attention. This is not meant to scare you, but it is the truth. Scheduling times and days that you are able to work out become a challenge. Use your support system to help you manage this time. Help will be needed and it is vital for you to make the appointments with yourself to slowly regain your strength, endurance, and your healthy lifestyle, overall. Add your resistance training days and cardiovascular days slowly. It may seem like a daunting task, but give yourself a few weeks and you will start to feel better and better each day. This is not just for your physical fitness, but also your mental well-being. Get yourself back to where you feel great, your little one deserves a healthy and happy Mommy!

Here is a recap for…

9 STEPS TO A HEALTHY PREGNANCY

(A) BEFORE

1. Discuss with physician your plan to have children. 6 months prior to pregnancy start a workout program that includes a pre-assessment of your health, resistance training, and cardiovascular training.

2. Research Fitness Professionals in your area who have obtained

an undergraduate degree minimum. Look for degrees in Exercise Science, Kinesiology, Biomechanics, etc. and also holding a Nationally Ranked Certification. Hire a Fitness Professional that you know you can trust and who can help you put together the best plan to build your muscular strength and endurance.

3. Start healthy habits of nutrition in your daily life. This is one of the most influential parts to ensure a successful pregnancy. Plan your workouts with your Fitness Professional so that you can be in the best health for you and your baby.

(B) DURING

4. Eat 6 small meals a day with lots of water. Just because you are carrying a child does not mean you are eating for two! With your doctor, determine the appropriate well-balanced nutrition plan that is appropriate for you. Keep your food simple and unprocessed as much as possible. This alone will help keep you at a healthy weight and feed the fetus appropriately.

5. Resistance training should be a minimum of 2 times per week with cardiovascular exercise 3 times per week. At first you will be able to exercise like you did before pregnancy and as you continue through your pregnancy you will want to monitor your heart rate (140-150 bpm maximum) and do not lie on your back after 16 weeks. By having good muscle endurance from exercise you are less likely to have back problems. Also, during delivery you will have the stamina and strength to push the fetus.

6. Your mental health is so important throughout your pregnancy. Your hormone levels will be up and down. With exercise you will release endorphins which will help enhance your mental state. It is natural that you will gain approximately 25-30 lbs. With appropriate exercise you will keep the weight gain under control, feel great, and decrease your risk for complications such as gestational diabetes, high blood pressure, etc.

(C) AFTER

7. It is important to listen to your body and your doctor at this time. If you delivered vaginally, 6 weeks is the normal amount of time to wait before exercising. With cesarean delivery, 8 weeks is the recommended time before starting back into exercise, but your doctor will tell you when you are ready. Start with walking for short durations and increase as you feel is appropriate, this will at least get you moving.

8. Your body is changing and your uterus is shrinking back to normal. If it is possible and in your plan, breast feeding is highly recommended. Formula cannot be compared to nutrients given to the baby through breast feeding, and will help you lose the baby weight faster.

9. As soon as you are released for exercise, you will need to start slowly and steadily. Your body has gone through many changes and you will find that you cannot exercise as fast and as much as you would like. Also, keep in mind, you need to ease back into abdominal and lower back exercises. Otherwise, you are encouraged to get back into your resistance training 2-3 times per week and cardiovascular exercise 2-3 days per week.

IN CONCLUSION

Plan your pregnancy and prepare your body to have the best pregnancy before, during, and after. If you are already pregnant and have not been exercising, it is not too late! Find a Fitness Professional you can trust and they will guide you to an appropriate program for both now and through the pregnancy.

As stated earlier, your core temperature will be elevated more while you are pregnant – which can lead to overheating and dehydration, so it is very important to keep hydrated and stay out of hot weather while exercising. After 16 weeks, do not lie on your back for any exercises as this can raise your heart rate and it can also decrease blood flow to the fetus. We also recommend wearing a heart rate monitor during any exercise. It is advisable to keep your heart rate below 140-150 beats per minute while exercising as well.

Enjoy this time of your life, embrace the changes to your body and take action! With your doctor, follow yourself to one of life's most rewarding experiences. Cherish this time and create a health and prosperous family!

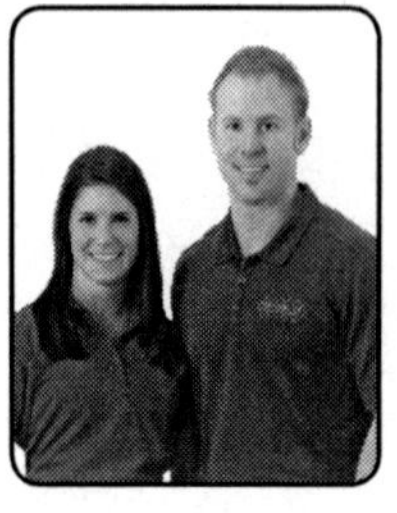

ABOUT ARIN & TONY

Arin Ralstin and Tony Lindauer, owners of Transformation Fitness and Wellness, a personal training studio, are leading providers of preventative health care in the Indianapolis market. They have transformed thousands of lives utilizing fitness and wellness strategies and continue to develop cutting- edge programs to address the growing healthcare crises. They have staffed qualified Fitness Professionals – who they continue to develop professionally and personally to change even more lives.

When Arin realized how she could change people's lives by motivating them, she sought out a Bachelor of Science degree in Exercise Science. When she received her first success story of a client no longer relying on arthritis medicine, she was hooked! Tony understood the science behind fitness and wellness because of his Master's of Science in Biomechanics, and became an advocate to educate clients on how to get the most out of their fitness. He has a passion to encourage all clients to challenge their bodies and take the tools from him and use them in their everyday life. One example was that of a gentleman who came in to Transformation Fitness and Wellness because of the extreme back pain that caused him the inability to stand up straight. Tony, who understands the value of living pain-free, was able to help the gentleman. In a matter of months, Tony had helped him strengthen his body, stretch properly, and now he walks everyday pain-free with improved posture!

With the growing 'epidemic' of unhealthy Americans, Arin and Tony are devoted to developing educated fitness and wellness solutions for all clients. When a person emails, calls, or walks through their door, they know they are going to be treated with integrity and a standard of care like no other. The Fitness Professionals at Transformation Fitness and Wellness must be educated, maintain a standard of personal health, and continue to develop themselves to provide 'best care' for each client. The compassion they have when they see the physical and emotional pain of a client, instantly makes them want to help alleviate that pain.

Arin, Tony and their staff are in the business of changing lives. They continue to do this every day and get the most gratification from their clients' testimonials. Each testimonial is another life changed forever. Come be transformed and be their next testimonial!

Contact:

Transformation Fitness and Wellness
www.tfwellness.com
support@tfwellness.com
317-927-9689

CHAPTER 16

KETTLEBELLS AND THE KEYS THAT MAKE THEM KING, PROVIDING SUPERIOR FITNESS FOR THE MASSES.

BY CHRIS GRAY

MY STORY

Over the last 13 years, I have been helping people regain control in their lives after many years of struggling with being overweight and out-of-shape. Throughout my time in the fitness industry, I have met with countless people who, after so many failures in accomplishing their goals, feel it is hopeless, and now believe nothing can be done. This story is a tragic one, and unfortunately I hear it more and more often every year.

In my early years as a fitness professional, I discovered what I believe is the greatest fallacy in the fitness industry today, and the number one reason for a client's failure to accomplish fitness and health goals. I sincerely believe that the fitness industry in general fails to do a good job providing accurate information and complete programs, which include all of the key elements to success that give clients the best chance to succeed.

In light of my discovery, my passion to provide a program that truly changes lives grew increasingly larger every year. I struggled with many failures myself to find the right methods and the right vehicle to deliver the best possible program to struggling clients. The program would have to provide all the keys elements to a successful transformation – not just pieces like my counterparts were doing.

Ten years later, I put the winning combination together with the opening of Punch Kettlebell Gym Dover, a personal training center with the sole purpose of getting people the bodies they have always wanted and the quality of life they truly deserve. At my training center, I have combined my experience and core values with the training methods of the kettlebell, finally giving people what they truly need to succeed.

WHY KETTLEBELLS...?

Kettlebells have now been vindicated as the king of cardio-fat burning and, in my opinion, have bridged the gap between strength training and cardiovascular training – making them the conditioning tool for the masses.

Scientific research has now shown us that kettlebells strip off unwanted body fat faster than any other form of exercise known today, getting twice the results in just half the time.

The research done by American Council on Exercise has shown us that after only a 20 minute kettlebell workout, subjects burned an average of 272 calories. Measurements revealed off the chart readings at 6.6 calories per minute which is equivalent to running at a 6 minute mile pace.

The success of the kettlebell can be credited to the fact that the entire body is being worked against gravity in unison at a rapid pace. When using kettlebells, there is a significant full body muscle activation not found in other types of training. It is because of this that you can do much more work in a shorter amount of time – producing rapid results.

One of the many advantages to kettlebell training making the method so unique is that the training teaches the body how to contend with a constantly changing center of gravity – replicating the same forces encountered in play, sport, and daily life. This is done by working the body across a wide variety of planes and angles just as we humans function in every day life. This is not an aspect of training that is addressed to this level in any traditional training method today, and why I chose kettlebells for my training center.

THE TRUTH ABOUT KETTLEBELLS

I have found in the last few years that when you say the word "kettlebell" a large number of people cringe or instantly discount their ability to use kettlebells. It seems that kettlebells have a certain level of fear surrounding them. It is unclear to me why this fear exists, but I can assure you there is nothing to fear!

My belief is that because kettlebells are different, and maybe outside someone's comfort zone, the perception is that kettlebells are not for them, when in fact the perception couldn't be more wrong. These dynamic tools are very user friendly, and after training hundreds of clients with them, I can tell you with certainty they can be used successfully by anyone of any age and fitness level.

A second reason why this fear may exist is because since kettlebells have moved into the mainstream and everyone is jumping on the bandwagon, there are more reported injuries while using kettlebells than in the recent past. The truth about kettlebells is yes, you can get injured using them, but your risks of injury are no more significant than any other training method out there today.

From my experience, I can tell you that in most cases the majority of the people who get injured using kettlebells are not using them correctly at the time of injury. Many people today attempt to do kettlebell training on their own at home with a store bought DVD and kettlebell set. Many are attending fitness centers that are holding kettlebell classes that are being guided by instructors who are not certified kettlebell instructors. A certified personal trainer is not good enough in the kettlebell world, your instructor must be a certified kettlebell instructor if you want to keep yourself safe.

The truth about kettlebells is this – yes, you can get hurt training with them as you can with any fitness program if form and technique are not held to the highest priority! I firmly believe that if you train with kettlebells using a certified instructor, your risk of injury is very low, and the level of success you can get in return is very high.

THE MISSING LINK

The missing link in kettlebell training today, which is responsible for most injuries, is foundation. As I stated earlier, I sincerely believe everyone can safely use kettlebells but the correct foundation must be built first, which is what a certified kettlebell instructor will teach you. I firmly believe that in almost every case when a novice picks up a kettlebell with no foundation, the techniques will be done wrong.

When first learning about kettlebells myself, I experienced many different programs and methods. I know now that I too was making mistakes, because I had no foundation to build on, then I found Art Of Strength. Once exposed to the AOS methods of kettlebell training it was clear to me that this was the program I needed for my training center. The entire focus of AOS methods are based on "foundation", the foundation is built using methods called "Corrective Strategies" and "Vintage Progressions". It is these methods that allow us to be sure the trainees have a good foundation first, and then systematically advance them as they are ready. To my knowledge, there is no other kettlebell training program that systemizes their training methods at this level.

The best advice I can give to those who are looking to experience this fantastic training tool, is be sure you have a certified kettlebell instructor – who will focus on building a solid foundation of strength and movement with a systemized approach. Do not make the mistake of so many and try training with kettlebells on your own. Invest in your health and learn the science behind the kettlebell methods and have fun doing it. Take it from me, the kettlebell can truly change your life if done the correct way.

SIX KEYS TO FITNESS SUCCESS

Now, as I stated earlier, having a complete fitness program to address all the key elements to success is essential, however this is often the weakest link in fitness today.

There really is no BIG secret to getting results with your health and fitness program. You do need, however, the right ingredients and a great coach. Because the real secret is your ability to implement the program on all levels. The real secret is taking action!

The reason people struggle to lose weight, get in shape, and make it last a lifetime is that they are lacking one or more of the following key ingredients. And leaving any of them out, is literally like trying to cook bread without an oven…

Here are the six key ingredients in no particular order:

1. **Strength Training** -You need strength training at least two days per week, and three is better. And this is serious strength training. Not the stuff you see other people doing at the gym. You need a strength training programs that cycles your training, builds muscle, and keeps your body fine-tuned like an athlete. No, you don't have to be young or be an athlete like the ones you see on TV. But you do have to approach the process in the same way and challenge yourself the way they do – to be successful.

2. **Cardiovascular Training** – You need cardiovascular exercise every day for a total of at least 150 minutes per week. No exceptions! No excuses. And no circuit training for goodness sake. Sorry ladies, Curves® doesn't cut it!

3. **Nutrition** – You must, must, must… eat 5-6 balanced meals throughout the day, take your vitamins, and stop eating junk food. Eating every 3 hours will control your metabolism and blood glucose which is not only essential for accomplishing your fitness goals but is also very important in the prevention of diabetes and other significant health problems. And don't worry, when you're eating right, all the junk food won't hold any power over you anymore, because you'll 'feel a ton better' and won't crave it anymore.

4. **Accountability** – This is a biggie for me!!! We know by ex-

perience that being accountable to someone will keep you on-track long term, and will be responsible for you being 50% more successful.

5. **Expert Guidance** – A coach will give the foundation needed to succeed, a plan of action that you can follow, and the motivational support required for success.

6. **Support** – A support structure in the form of programming, testing, coaches and the rest of the community of people who are on the same path will be essential for your success.

I want to strongly emphasize that you need all six of these things working for you to maximize your results. What happens most often is that people have only one or two of them going and then wonder why it's not working.

The other problem is that they are often not working hard enough during their exercise, and this can really hinder progress. That's another great reason to have a trainer and a coach who can push you.

TOP TWO "WHAT NOT TO DO" FOR FITNESS SUCCESS

I have heard these words many times over the years! "…I'm not hungry"!

Here's is the deal…when you are trying to achieve a lean fit body, it doesn't matter if you are hungry or not, you must eat every three hours. From the time you wake up in the morning till the time you go to bed at night, you are on the clock…literally! In fact, many of my clients frequently set an alarm on their phone, watch, or computer to remind them that it is time to eat again. Sound crazy…???

The key to fat loss is increasing the metabolism! The only safe way to do that is eating small meals frequently throughout the day. I frequently use the analogy of the engine in your car, if you want your car to go faster, you step on the gas which gives the engine more fuel causing the car to speed up. Well the metabolism works the same way! If you want the metabolism to speed up, you must increase the amount of fuel you are giving the body by eating frequent small healthy meals all through the day – which causes the metabolism to speed up!

Some may say "You're crazy…I'm trying to lose weight and you want me to eat more!" YES, that is correct! Diets and calorie restriction do not work, in fact its the worse thing you could possibly do and you will never achieve long term success if you choose to take that path. Let me emphasize that you are eating "healthy" meals every three hours, not junk food!

Please understand that 90% of your results comes from what you put in your mouth, so if you truly want success and have total control over your long term health, then you absolutely must educate yourself or invest in a coach and commit to a healthy nutrition program that you can maintain for life!

If there is one thing that over the last 10 years has been my biggest headache, 'hands down', its the argument that scale weight means nothing! On a daily basis I have to remind clients that when you step on that scale, the number you see is relative and therefore not an accurate measure of results.

The simple fact of the matter is if you are doing everything right, your scale weight will not change much, at least in the beginning of your weight-loss journey. What I mean is as you begin taking steps to improve your health and increase metabolism by weight training and eating six small meals throughout the day you will begin gaining muscle. This is a necessary process if you want results!

So what occurs is, as you are losing inches and body fat you are also gaining necessary muscle mass – which offsets your losses on the scale, giving the appearance that you are not getting results! Remember that muscle weighs more than fat, and that in fact is what you see when you step on that scale.

I ask everyone the same question when they come to me with this question. Have you lost inches...? Do you feel better...? Has your strength and endurance improved…? Has your clothing become looser…?

In almost every case the answers to all of those questions are "Yes", however they always are followed by the word "BUT". No buts,… if you answered yes to the above questions then you are doing exactly what you need to do in order to achieve results! Yes the weight will come down eventually as long as you are doing everything correct, but it takes some time.

The key to getting the weight off and keeping it off is a safe, slow loss in body fat, as you gain new lean body mass to stimulate metabolism and give you that "tone" everyone wants. It's the people who want a quick weight loss using some fad diet program or diet pills that lose all that weight very quickly, then, before you know it, gain it all back! Its the people who dedicate themselves to a lifestyle change and put in the hard work and long term commitment that will succeed every time and enjoy their new body for the rest of their lives.

The big point I want everyone to come away with here is that the scale is not an accurate way of measuring results. You could easily be discouraged if you only looked at the scale weight, and many people fall into this trap!

Have a professional take all the necessary measurements to reveal your true results, because if you're doing things correctly, the muscle you gain will offset the scale weight giving the illusion that you're not getting results. You must throw the scale away and measure body fat percentage and lean muscle mass to correctly measure progress.

I wish you the best in your fitness journey. I hope what we talked about here today will help you in finally accomplishing your goals.

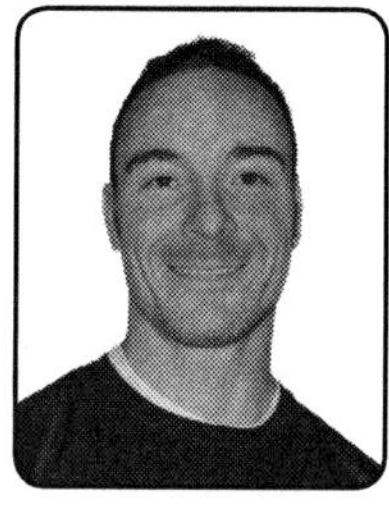

ABOUT CHRIS

Chris has been in the fitness industry for over a decade now, where he has made his mark as one of Delaware's top trainers and club owners. His very unique kettlebell training center is literally changing lives using techniques and equipment never before seen by most.

After years of witnessing people struggle every day to lose weight and get in shape, Chris realized that most gyms and fitness programs set people up to fail right from the start – by not providing them with all of the key elements needed to achieve success. It's the failure to provide these tools that result in most people failing to accomplish their fitness and health goals.

At Punch Kettlebell Gym based in Dover Delaware, Chris and his team provide all the essential tools that most programs miss and offer guaranteed results! His highly-trained team prides themselves with a mission to be the best part of each member's day everyday! We will over deliver a 'wow' experience beyond anything each member has ever been a part of, providing all the key elements of success to each of our members to ensure their successful lifestyle change.

Chris Gray, the owner of Punch is a graduate of Polytech High School, and a graduate of Cecil Community College. He now serves full time as a firefighter/paramedic for a department in Maryland. Chris is a competitive body builder and a former semi pro football player. He has also competed nationally in 3 World Championships with an elite team of professionals in the Scott Firefighter Combat Challenge. Chris is an AFPA certified personal trainer, strength coach, and an Art Of Strength kettlebell instructor.

You can contact Chris Gray with questions by email at: chris@punchgym.com

To receive free fitness reports and newsletters from Chris, go to:
www.FreeFitnessDownloads.com

To sign up for a free consultation and discovery workout with Chris, go to:
www.PunchGymFitness.com

Company Websites:
www.PunchGymDover.com
www.DelawareBootCamps.com

CHAPTER 17

TAKING YOUR TRAINING TO THE NEXT LEVEL

BY JASON LONG

PROGRAM DESIGN

Since my wife and I have been married we've made several trips to Boston from our hometown in Buffalo, each trip planned out differently. Our first road trip to Boston resembled the journey an amateur athlete or fitness enthusiast is on to reach their desired destination or goals. We actually had a plan, a map from a local travel service that paved the way to Boston. Just follow the highlighted route and before long we'll be there…right? Well…sort of. Although that map served as a guide, like many workouts from books and magazines do for most people, it never accounted for our specific situation – what we needed right then. In other words, it couldn't accurately predict or address our specific needs at that time. We were moving in the right direction but with a lot of unexpected bumps in the road.

As circumstances changed, our journey remained the same because our map did not offer flexibility and allow for modifications based on new circumstances. Sound familiar? You started a workout because it either looked good to you or was recommended by someone else. BUT, that workout never asked you, "Hey, what is your body already used to, based on what workout you've done the last few months?" or …"What is the time frame that you would like to achieve your goal?" When you hit a roadblock or plateau, you just keep pushing, just like we just kept driving. And… well, that's ridiculous.

The idea is to train smart, not just train hard. The last couple trips we've made to Boston was with a GPS. Talk about coasting! If we wanted the fastest route that avoided detours we had it. Or if we preferred the cheapest route, that was also available. It offered turn-by-turn directions with a lot less work on our end. It was a more efficient and less stressful method of getting to our destination. Your workout program should be just like our trip with a GPS. It should be very efficient and specific to you and your goals, and it should change over time based on the present circumstances. It's not rocket science. Many people give up on a certain goal or exercise routine altogether, because they just didn't have all the right tools to create more effective change.

The bottom line is you want **RESULTS**, and you should get them. Although there are a number of variables and other factors that go into effective program design, you can use the acronym **RESULTS** to remember and implement several of them. **R** stands for **reps** and **ROM** (range of motion). **E** stands for **exercise selection** and **exercise order**. **S** stands for **sets**. **U** stands for **undulating**. **L** stands for **load** or intensity. **T** stands for **time** or rest. **S** stands for **speed** and **specificity**.

Be sure to write down the acrostic **RESULTS** vertically on a sheet of paper and what each letter stands for. Then write down what you've done over the past couple months for each of those letters. You should start to see a pattern (i.e., always doing a similar rep range or movements with the same angles/ROM, speed, etc.).

REPS – **R**ep ranges will ultimately dictate the intensity level in which you are working. Assuming you are lifting for a RM (repetition maximum – total number of reps executed before complete fatigue) and only doing 1 rep (equivalent to the maximum amount of weight you can lift) vs. 20 reps, will have a completely different effect on your body. Working at different rep ranges will allow you to create a different stimulus for each range and therefore emphasize different goals. A rep range of 1-3 with a large emphasis on speed of movement is an explosive power range where 1-3RM and even 4-6RM will serve to promote increases in strength. All individuals can make significant increases in their strength at the 4-6RM range while those with more training experience will want to explore the true maximum effort range of 1-3RM for greater gains. A hypertrophic (muscle gain) rep range is typically between 8-10RM where muscular endurance is emphasized more with the higher rep ranges 14+. It is important to note that the body will adapt to any repetition range you give it within just a few exposures (workouts). This is why you don't want to do the same rep ranges all the time, or you will hit a plateau quickly and compromise results. For example, a fat loss goal may emphasize a rep range of 6-8 in one workout, 14-18 in another, and 11-13 in a third workout and you may rotate those rep ranges with different workouts each week for a month. Because a rep range of 8-10 might be best for muscular hypertrophy, that does not mean it is not also effective for fat loss.

ROM – **R**ange of motion, or the joint angle of an exercise will dictate if the body receives a new stimulus or the same one it's used to. Take the most widely used exercise – bench press. If you always perform this exercise with a full ROM and at the same angle (i.e. elbow level with the chest) then your body will consistently use the same muscular recruitment pattern to complete that movement. The take home message here is change it up. At some point only go down halfway, or go down all the way but only come halfway up. Change the joint angle so maybe your elbow comes just below your chest or just above. This will create a new stimulus and elicit further change in your body. The change you should make will be dictated by your goals.

EXERCISE – **E**xercise selection and exercise order are two very simple variables that, when changed regularly, will improve results and prevent boredom. Exercises, in my opinion, should be changed every 2-6 weeks on average, especially when there is a goal of improved athletic performance. More advanced individuals may need to rotate exercises more frequently because they adapt quicker. Once full adaptation takes place, the body will no longer respond to what you are giving it. Less experienced individuals may use the same exercises for a couple months before it's no longer effective at creating change.

Every exercise should be grouped into a movement complex. All horizontal pushing exercises (i.e. Barbell Bench press - flat, incline, decline; Dumbbell Bench press - flat, incline, decline; Standing cable press,) would constitute a movement complex. Every month you would rotate through a new exercise within each given movement complex to ensure you are still working that muscle group, but are changing the stimulus enough to continue to create change (i.e., month 1: Flat Db Bench; month 2: Standing cable press; etc.).

Exercise order is really quite simple…change the order of the exercises in your workout. Exercises performed later in your workout will be affected by fatigue from those exercises performed earlier. You can use this principle to structure your workout based on your underlying goal. If you want to improve your squat strength, then don't perform your leg exercises at the tail end of your workout when your energy tank is running low and your performance will be comprised.

SETS – The number of **S**ets performed in a workout will also affect the stimulus the body receives. A goal of hypertrophy and fat loss will typically require more sets whereas a goal of increased strength may require fewer sets but performed at a much higher intensity (1-3RM). Volume is an important variable to note here. Volume is calculated by multiplying your sets times reps times weight lifted (sets x reps x weight). Oftentimes, changing your volume will overload your body just enough to create that change you're looking for. To create change, you must overload your body by either changing the load (intensity and volume) above what you're used to, or changing the exercise. For an easy but effective change in your routine, try focusing on several new set and rep ranges for the next several weeks.

UNDULATION – **U**ndulation is defined in the Merriam-Webster dictionary as having a wavelike motion or appearance; to rise and fall in pitch and volume. This is how your workout should look. Technically speaking, it is called *flexible non-linear periodization*. The primary rep range utilized for a four-week period will be based upon your goal, with other rep ranges infused throughout each workout. The first couple weeks may contain workouts of relatively higher sets and lighter loads, while the last couple weeks may decrease in volume but the intensity is significantly increased. The rest time between sets and exercises should fluctuate slightly over the course of the month, but may be slightly shorter as the program progresses and you become more conditioned. Rest times should increase for those workouts containing high intensity and increased load (heavy weight with low reps) – to allow for greater recovery. The speed of movement as a whole may be relatively quick, with a slight emphasis on some isometric holds at the end range of the movements during select workouts (bottom of a bench press, squat, etc.). **Remember…It is change that creates more change!**

If the same load (intensity), reps, exercises and volume are performed over a long enough period of time, that individual will experience accommodation, which states that the response of a biological object to a constant stimulus decreases over time. The objective of any workout regimen is to provide the correct stimulus (workout) with the result being fitness gain or performance improvement by way of adaptation. This is why it is beneficial to do the same exercises over a period of time in order to allow adaptation and positive change to occur. Once the body has adapted to a particular movement or exercise, you then modify the program to continue to make progress.

Lastly, a well-thought out program will account for, and meet the needs of, day-to-day changes and fluctuations in energy levels as a result of inadequate sleep, poor nutrition, mental fatigue and general physical fatigue. Though Monday might be an all-out maximum effort day of 1-3RM or high intensity cardiovascular intervals, if you have any fatigue present your workout intensity will suffer. If your goal is to increase strength, but you are fatigued, you may not push hard enough or use the loads necessary to improve your strength.

LOAD – Load or intensity is based on the weight you are lifting which will dictate the reps you are able to perform. The heaviest of all weights (maximum effort – 1RM) will only allow you to complete one rep before you completely fatigue. There is a direct correlation with intensity and load. Greater loads (or weight) will increase intensity whereas lighter loads will decrease intensity. By consistently changing your repetition ranges, assuming you are working to fatigue, you are also altering your intensity. Keep in mind that you can change your volume through the load or weight you lift as well. Damage to muscle tissue and the resultant recovery of that tissue is what leads to change. The two ways to damage muscle tissue are through load or chemical damage. The rest time between sets will have the greatest effect on chemical damage.

TIME – Time or rest between sets and exercises can significantly influence your level of fatigue, the total work you do in a period of time, and chemical damage to your muscle tissue. Work capacity (the ability to do more in the same or less time) can be improved by decreasing the amount of time between sets and exercises, while also increasing muscular endurance and fitness capacity. Keeping intensity relatively high through explosive lifts and other key movements that place a great demand on the body, with minimal rest periods, can significantly increase EPOC (excess post-exercise oxygen consumption). EPOC is one of the main goals for any effective fat loss program. Taking in more oxygen by working harder with minimal rest periods will significantly increase the amount of calories burned during and after the workout, therefore increasing fat loss.

Rest periods of sixty seconds or less between sets are ideal for hypertrophic goals to create chemical damage (often felt through the "burn" you feel during strength exercises). Decreased rest periods will also allow your body to improve its muscular endurance through buffering and clearing lactic acid more efficiently (what causes the burn) so you don't experience the burn/fatigue as quickly and can handle more work. Longer rest periods of 2-3 minutes or more should be used for those individuals looking to increase their level of strength. This will better allow them to recover between sets so they can maintain their intensity levels without fatiguing prematurely – due to fatigue from inadequate rest.

SPEED – **S**peed or tempo is yet another variable that can be manipulated regularly to create further change. Speed or tempo is simply the speed at which you lift the weight through its desired range of motion. The most significant muscle damage occurs through lengthening muscular contractions or eccentric contractions. So, instead of lowering a barbell at a normal speed in a bench press, you might take 3, 4, or 5 seconds to lower it all the way down, which will significantly increase the intensity and alter the stimulus your body receives through that particular exercise. Fast concentric contractions, quickly lifting the weight up in a bench press or isometric contractions where you would hold the weight typically at the end range of motion (i.e. bottom of the bench press), both can provide enough of a stimulus in and of themselves – to further create positive change. For goals of explosive power or fat loss, lifting a weight with great speed, as in a clean or snatch, can significantly increase the demand on the body, and therefore the total amount of calories burned resulting in a greater amount of lean body mass over a period of time.

Whatever your goal is, you can start by making some modifications to your current program based on the acronym RESULTS. Remember that the body will always adapt to exactly what you do, so start by changing your program and doing something different with the goal of making the most amount of change with the least amount of effort. The key phrase there is “the most with the least.” For example, you may only need to increase your usual number of sets by two, instead of jumping up to four extra sets to create change. This will allow the opportunity for a greater number of progressions over time, leading to more consistent results. It must be progressive and systematic – especially for an athletic performance goal. Results are always within your grasp – it’s just a matter of consistency, patience, having a vast enough toolbox, and knowing how to use each tool to create effective change.

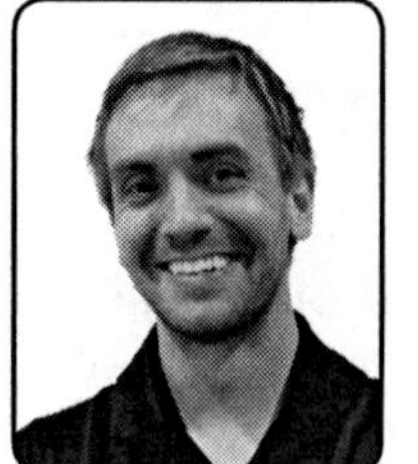

ABOUT JASON

Jason Long, President and Founder of TREO Sports & Fitness, is a successful business owner, having helped 100's of clients through a results-driven training system for both athletes and fitness enthusiast.

Jason founded his company in 2008, after spending 6 years working at various health and sport clubs in California and New York. He currently holds a certification as a certified personal trainer through NASM and a certified strength and conditioning specialist through the NSCA. He returned to Buffalo to complete his Master's degree in Exercise Science in order to pursue his dream to open an athletic performance and fitness studio. He recently completed his level 3 certification through Z Health and plans to continue his educational background.

After spending years in competitive athletics, Jason realized his goal to provide a comprehensive training system to local athletes that would dramatically increase their overall performance and level of play. Jason's performance training system has helped dozens of athletes significantly improve various skills necessary for high level athletic performance and consistently improve their vertical jump 2-4.5" inches in just 8 training sessions while also seeing as much as a 4/10 of a second drop in the 40 yd dash in just 4 training sessions.

On the fitness end, he realized that selling memberships to a club wasn't the answer to client results, but instead an individual and personalized plan that included injury prevention, proper recovery, fat loss and muscle building tools would help them achieve their goals. Jason has spent years researching, developing, and integrating various methods of training to consistently improve the TREO training system. He, along with his staff, has achieved superb results with each client, time and time again.

To learn more about TREO Sports & Fitness and Jason Long, and how you can receive free special reports, please visit www.TREOSportsFitness.com

CHAPTER 18

GET OUT OF YOUR BOX TO MAKE FITNESS FUN

BY ERIK PEACOCK

People face many obstacles when it comes to fitness that have to deal with motivation, self discipline, and just plain knowing how to put together an effective plan. However, one factor is often overlooked by some of the best personal trainers. That factor is BOREDOM. Yes, fitness can be boring. (There, I admitted it.) I just hope the 'personal training mafia' doesn't scoop me up, tie kettlebells to my legs and throw me into a lake. It's true we get caught up with sets, reps, bodyfat percentages, heart rate training zones and bodyfat percentages. Aaaagggh!!! It drives me crazy sometimes.

Why is it so many fitness routines remind me of a gift opening the day after a wedding? You feel you have to go, but being a part of it pales in comparison to sorting your sock drawer. (Now I'll probably have the 'bride mafia' after me.)

Anyway, let me get to the point about this chapter. In order for someone to stick to fitness as a lifelong habit, it needs be fun and enjoyable for it to be a priority. Think about other things you enjoy, like watching your favorite TV show, golf, coffee with friends, or playing poker. I know many people who do these things regularly. Why is that? Because they are enjoyable, fun, and help people connect.

So why can't fitness be more like this?

It can, and I'm going to give some examples of how we make it fun at our studio. You see, we believe that people don't just buy personal training from us, they are really buying an experience. Think about it – they get up, drag themselves into a job they hate, work in a high stress environment all day, sit in traffic, and then go home to deal with the demands their families put on them – from cooking to running kids around. However, a few times per week they get to go into a place where they laugh, sweat, play and feel good about what they've accomplished when they leave. You see, to us it's more important that a client of ours leaves our facility feeling better than when they came in. It's more important than how many calories they burned or how much weight they lifted. We believe clients who have a super positive and uplifting experience will be lifelong clients. We want to be the highlight of their day, not just another mundane task on the list next to ...'pick up dry cleaning.'

For example, one of the things I have done with my group workouts is to 'theme them out'. For instance, one day was Navy Seal Training Day, one day was Football Day, and one day was Counter Terrorism Day.

On Navy Seal Day, I did things like having them crawl under "barbed wire" which was really rubber tubing strung across the studio. I had them "swim" across the studio on the ab dolly which was really good for training the upper back and core. They did "weapons training" by doing some great swinging core and upper body movements with an Olympic bar.

On Football Day, they completed the drills I did when I played football. Yes, I modified them but they were a great change up for the participants. They got to smack the dummy, bear crawl and go out for pass patterns. We have also done the dreaded updowns, where you have to jog, drop to the ground, and then get up (a killer cardio exercise), where they have to chant something silly while doing them. One time I made them chant in unison, marine-style: "I love hairbands from the 80s." (Yes, I'm a fan of the hard rock of the 80s). On Counter Terrorism Day, they got to hit, kick, throw and punch things. One time I even put a picture of myself on the heavy bag to motivate the class to hit it harder.

The best thing was that everyone worked, had fun, and laughed as well. That pretty much sums it up – work hard/play hard at the same time.

One of our big pushes lately is to get clients 'out of the box' of going to the gym. A few years back, collectively, as a staff, we came up with the Jumpstart Challenge. This contest required people partner up with someone. The contest ran for 10 weeks and participants earned points by doing regular strength, cardio, and flexibility workouts as well as food journals. However, if they wanted big time points they had to complete fitness challenges such as doing a rock climbing wall, mountain biking one of the areas challenging courses, or doing our "banding together" class – which had them work their whole body with just rubber tubing. Many of them found they really enjoyed these activities – which they would not have tried had it not been for the Jumpstart contest. One client, who was deathly afraid of heights, topped the rock climbing wall four times. Another one told me after doing the mountain bike course for the first time she was "scared —-tless," but had fun at the same time – like being on a roller coaster. To me, the best thing was seeing people accomplish things they never thought they could.

Another offering we added that really made fitness fun was our fitness adventure retreats. Here is where we had to be super creative, because people were spending a whole weekend with us, not just one hour. So we had to come up with some good stuff to keep them engaged. Well, I'm happy to say they have been a huge success, not because they were great workouts, but because they were fun for the participants.

Here are a few of the highlights that participants really liked:

The Friday Adventure hike/trail run. We had participants wear their heart rate monitors and took them down a hiking course in one of our State Parks. We mixed in jogging, power walking as well as stations like pushups on a fallen tree, and power rock throws into the lake. Trust me, this cardio work was more intensive than level 20 on the stepmill.

Playground Bootcamp. One of our most talented trainers created a complete bootcamp circuit utilizing a kids playground, swings and sand volleyball courts. People did things like hang from the bars, do 'agilities' through the swings, and crawl up the slide.

Amazing Race Lake City. The town we were in was Lake City, Minnesota, which is a small town of about 5,000 people situated on the Mississippi river. It was very scenic, surrounded by beautiful bluffs. We decided to mimic the show "Amazing Race" and set up stations where teams of two would have to complete a challenge and then answer a trivia question before moving to the next station. We had set up a course all through the town. The challenges varied from climbing up the rocks from the river (not as bad as it sounds), to dragging a weighted sled through the sand. Yeah. I know it sounds bad, but everyone was done in less than 40 minutes and we had many different levels of fitness taking part.

The retreats really showed me that people are looking for new experiences and enjoy accomplishing something other than making it three miles on the treadmill.

Alright, I've given you some examples of things we do to get 'out of the box' with our clients, but I also want to give you some great tips on how to make your own fitness fun and keep it fresh.

HERE ARE SIX TIPS TO KEEP FITNESS FUN AND NOT FORCED

1. THINK OF YOURSELF LIKE AN ATHLETE

Serious athletes train year round. They might only be in one sport, but they plan to train so they peak right when they start their season, maintain during the season and recover afterwards. Why can't you take this approach? We like to get our clients to think of themselves as athletes in training, so they have more purpose when going to the gym instead of 'just to work out'. For example, a client might have a big ski trip planned for the mountains in the winter, so we prep them with specific phases and exercises designed to help them be quick, reactive and agile – so they are prepared to deal with moguls, wild terrain, and crazy snowboarders. The same client might want to play golf during the summer, so we start the golf phase after the ski trip. You get the picture. Everyone's different, but treating them all like athletes gives them more purpose and makes them feel 'more cool' when it comes to training.

2. FIND OR CREATE THE ENVIRONMENT YOU NEED TO ENERGIZE YOU

Too many people choose a gym just for its proximity, but it has the atmosphere of a funeral parlor; or they try to work out at home thinking they can save a few bucks, but that great machine they bought on the Home Shopping Network seems to be used more for drying clothes than exercise. Find a place that has some energy. I know too many people who join a gym to save a few bucks, but end up never going because it has no life. Find something that matches you. I like old dungeons with free weights and 'heavy metal' music blasting, but this is probably not for the 60 year-old woman trying to reduce her back pain and lose some weight.

3. JOIN A GROUP

The big move in the personal training field is from individual to small group training. I believe this is for two reasons. Number one is the economy, as it is typically cheaper to work out in a group than by yourself. The other is that groups are more fun period. You make new friends, develop camaraderie, and keep each other both accountable and motivated. Our group training most times is more lively. Even though these people are working hard, they still seem to give us as well as each other a hard time about the music, hairstyles, outfits or whatever they can think up. My point is the dynamic here is 'fun and lively.' So find an exercise group of people you connect with or create one of your own with your friends. Just look at how many running, biking and hiking clubs there are out there. It's just as much about the social part as the exercise part.

4. TRY NEW THINGS AT LEAST ONCE A QUARTER

Mix it up often to avoid boredom. Here is one thing I like to do and it's made my exercise much more enjoyable. I pick something once a quarter to try out. I used to avoid mountain biking, thinking it would ruin my regular workouts because I was stuck 'in my box'. When I finally tried it, it was like 'crack', I was hooked. It is now a staple of my cardio routine and other people who I've introduced it to now love it as much as I do. Had I stayed in my box, I would have missed out on what is now my favorite outdoor activity. Not only do I get a good workout, but

I get to experience our awesome nature parks firsthand and time goes by fast. Whatever your fitness level, there are tons of things out there, from kayaking to Zumba. I'll bet there is something you haven't tried that you would love.

5. CHANGE YOUR ROUTINE OFTEN

Still don't get how people can go to the gym and do the same routine day after day, week after week, year after year. YAWN! YAWN! You want to keep things fresh and mix it up often (every 4-6 weeks). You can even do hybrid weeks, where one day is a strength day, one day is bootcamp, and maybe one day is kettlebells day. Whatever it is, change it up frequently, or you will find yourself going through the motions – which is just a step away from quitting altogether.

6. USE GOOD MUSIC MIXES

I think the I-Pod could be the greatest invention ever. It amazes me how effective creating playlists to match workouts is. Hopefully, you have an MP3 player or an iPod; if not, buy one. Create some 'killer mixes' that give you the boost you need to get through a challenging workout. Many workout facilities tend to play contemporary music, which is really another word for 'elevator' music, so use your own if this is the case. Hey, if 'elevator' music is your thing, then stick with it.

So what's the point of this whole chapter? No, I'm not telling you that you need to run through the woods and scale a rockwall to have fun. What I hope you'll get out of this chapter is that fitness shouldn't just be relegated to the confines of a gym. Get outside, try new things and don't get caught up in urban myths such as "I have to run to lose weight", or "all I have to do is 20 sets of bench press to get that muscular look I want." There are many paths which lead to lifelong fitness and we don't all have to be on the same one. *The important thing to remember is that in order to make fitness a part of your lifestyle for the long term, it has to be something you feel you want to do, not have to do.*

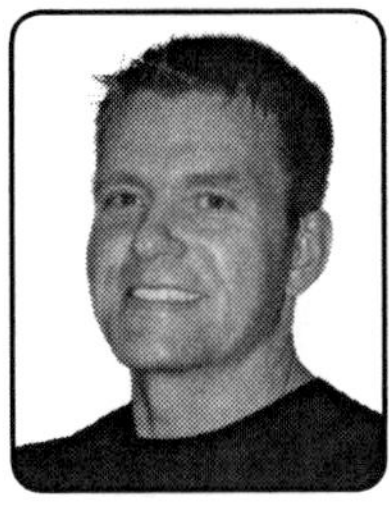

ABOUT ERIK

Erik Peacock has spent over 16 years in the fitness industry, molding and crafting his personal training system – using his own creativity as well as the education he has received from top experts in the industry. He is considered an expert in weight loss, sport specific training, corrective exercise and nutrition. Currently, he holds two accredited personal training certifications; the first is from the National Academy Of Sports Medicine (NASM) as a performance enhancement specialist, and the other is from The National Strength And Conditioning Association (NSCA) as a certified personal trainer.

His current company, Puravida Fitness, was founded in 2005. The name came from the concept "Puravida" – a word from Costa Rica which simply means 'a zest for life'. He focuses on applying this concept in his business by helping people with "life specific" training and nutrition programs. They are customized to help them get the most out of life and enjoy it to the fullest, through exercise and positive lifestyle changes.

He is based in Lakeville, Minnesota, which is a suburb of Minneapolis in the Twin Cities area –where he was been featured on local radio shows and television.

To learn more about Erik Peacock, his business Puravida Fitness, and how you can get his newsletters and special reports jammed with valuable fitness and nutrition tips, just go to: www.puravidafitness.com or call him direct at 952-220-2448.

CHAPTER 19

THE SECRET TO IGNITING YOUR METABOLISM FOR MAXIMUM FAT BURNING RESULTS

– HOW TO USE SIMPLE BODY WEIGHT AND DUMBBELL EXERCISES ALONG WITH SHORT, FUN, FULL BODY WORKOUTS TO QUICKLY SCULPT YOUR ARMS, ABS AND LEGS IN RECORD TIME!

BY ERIC GELDER

Everyone wants a faster metabolism so they can eat whatever they want (within reason), and still have a shapely set of arms, a pair of long lean muscular legs, and abs 'to die for'. The problem with most exercise routines is that they don't deliver the type of fat loss results you're looking for.

Whether you're a stay-at-home mom or the CEO of a Fortune 500 company, we're all pressed for time and that stacks the cards against us from the very beginning. That's why you need to have an effective workout plan in place to maximize your workout time to its fullest extent. If you're going to use exercise to shape your body, which you must, then it only makes sense to do it effectively and derive the greatest impact on your metabolism from performing it properly.

THREE METABOLISM BOOSTING WORKOUT TIPS

1. PERFORM FULL BODY COMPOUND EXERCISES – NOT ISOLATION EXERCISES.

Compound exercises are exercises that utilize several muscle groups across multiple joints, as compared to isolation movements that only require you to use one muscle group and one joint at a time.

When choosing exercises to perform in your workout, select big calorie burning exercise like variations of exercises such as Squats, Jumps, Deadlifts, Swings, Lunges, Presses, Rows, Push-Ups, Pull-Ups, Dips and Full body plank-based abdominal exercises.

Not only do these full body exercises increase your caloric expenditure far beyond what isolation exercises do, but they allow you to decrease your workout time, allowing you to get in and out as quickly and efficiently as possible, with a minimum time investment.

2. INCREASE YOUR STRENGTH

When you're exercising to get stronger, your body is primed for maximum metabolism increases. When you're stronger, you're able to perform more exercise in the same or even less time than it normally would take you. So accomplishing more exercise in less time means better fat loss results along with a greater increase in your fitness capacity. Both allow you to attain maximum body composition changes.

Always continue striving to get stronger by doing more in less time, using more resistance for your exercises or performing more repetitions of each exercise. That's the reason it's called Progressive Resistance Strength Training.

3. PERFORM INTERVALS

Intervals are not only more time-effective than longer cardio sessions, but more results-effective.

One thing to always keep in mind with exercise is that the more challenging it is, the more your metabolism is having to work to adapt to that particular exercise session. The more challenging the adaptation, the more effective it is at assisting you with your fat loss goals.

Cruising around your neighborhood for a five mile jog is not only hard on your joints, but less effective for losing fat than performing sprints on a track, shuttle runs in a park, high-incline power walking intervals on a treadmill or other interval-based training. The longest you'd want to make an interval for the purpose of effectively increasing your metabolism is 120 seconds, and more often 60 seconds or less works even better because of the sustainability of your effort.

It's not really about the "time" *per se*, it's more about the effort you put forth, so keep that in mind. You can either go long and easy or short and hard – with short and hard being where the maximum results are going to be. You should be looking for the biggest bang for the amount of time involved, and intervals are a superior form of activity for fat loss because of that.

Do you know how to structure your exercise program for maximum results in minimum time?

Let's look at what will give you the most "bang for your buck" because that's what we all want. To spend the least amount of time exercising and for it to deliver the biggest fat loss response from it that we can get. To do that, we're going to use a specific type of interval exercise. That type of exercise is *Resistance Based Interval Training*. When looking for the gold standard in fat loss exercise, resistance based interval training will provide you with the biggest bang for your time and your metabolism.

IMPORTANT POINT:

Resistance training (weight training) provides you with the biggest metabolic effect. Most tend to believe that resistance exercise is only for building larger muscles and getting stronger, but often don't realize the importance resistance exercise has on eliciting a very powerful fat loss response from their body. If your goal is to lose body fat and transform your body into the firm, fit and fabulous body you desire, then resistance exercise should be 'front and center' in your fat loss program.

In order to maximize your metabolism, you need to have muscle. Coincidentally, any form of long cardio training sessions are counterproductive to accomplishing that goal. Too much exercise volume starts to impede progress from the excessive elevation of the catabolic adrenal "stress" hormone cortisol. In order to mitigate that, we'll alternate your resistance interval training on an every other day basis and steer clear of long exercise sessions, which lead to less muscle and therefore a less than optimal metabolism.

Let me provide you with a quick example of this in action to illustrate my point.

Name: Mary Smith
Body Weight: 180 lbs
Body Fat: 30%
Lean Body Mass: 126 lbs
Body Fat Mass: 54 lbs

Mary is a typical forty year old mother. She has three young children under the age of ten and she's finally hit her breaking point. Mary decides she's had it with being thirty pounds overweight, feeling unhealthy, and not having a positive body image. Mary's choice to reverse this scenario, gain back her self-confidence and look like she did before having her three children is as follows:

Her method is to do lots of long cardio sessions and reduce her total calories to non-sustaining levels. Let's take a look at Mary's results after her twelve weeks, and see what she was able to accomplish using her long cardio and nutritionally-deficient eating plan.

Name: Mary Smith
Body Weight: 160 lbs
Body Fat: 27%
Lean Body Mass: 117 lbs
Body Fat Mass: 43 lbs

After twelve weeks of being consistent with her aggressive weight loss plan, Mary sees that she's lost 20 lbs or about two-thirds of her original weight loss goal and feels like she's succeeded. Although the scale shows she's down twenty pounds, she's left to wonder why her clothes aren't a looser fit from all her weight loss.

If we dig a little deeper into her results, we can see where she went wrong. Mary ended up losing 20 lbs with 9 lbs of that from her lean muscle and 11 lbs from her body fat. She actually lost almost half her scale weight loss (45%) from lean muscle and the remainder from her body fat. Not good. Since we talked earlier about muscle being the driving force for your metabolism to optimally function for fat loss, we can gather that she's reduced her ability to burn body fat, and will lose even more lean muscle if she continues going down that path for much longer.

Mary's total drop in body fat percentage was actually a paltry 3% after three hard months of long cardio sessions and restrictive eating. With your metabolism being dictated by the amount of lean muscle you have on your body, you can see her metabolism's effectiveness has been severely reduced. Soon it will cause her to plateau with her weight loss efforts because of her inability to burn calories effectively.

Now that her body has less lean muscle, her eating habits will dramatically affect her ability to store calories once she decides she can no longer sustain her restrictive nutritional approach to weight loss. Plain and simple, she will now gain weight back at a faster rate once her normal calorie levels are resumed because she has less muscle on her body. This is true even if her exercise volume remains the same.

Therein lies our reason for using resistance-based exercise to maintain and ultimately increase your lean muscle mass while losing body fat at the same time. Through the above illustration you can see the relationship you have between your muscles, your metabolism and the results you achieve from your fat loss program. To be successful at transforming your body from soft, weak and unhealthy, you must understand that the efficient way is through the proper use of a well-planned resistance-based exercise program with a "twist". That twist is the addition of intervals to your resistance-training program with three simple steps.

THREE STEPS FOR A PERFECT FAT LOSS WORKOUT

Step #1 – Dynamic Activity Warm Up
Step #2 – Resistance Exercise Interval Workout
Step #3 – Static Stretching Cool Down and Recovery

STEP #1: DYNAMIC ACTIVITY WARM-UP (5-10 MINUTES)

Your warm-up should not be taken lightly. It's imperative that you warm-up properly to ensure that your body is prepared for the exercise you're about to do. By warming up, you will increase your core body temperature, increase the viscosity of your joints, increase your heart rate and be mentally ready for the exercise session to come. This all lends itself to the reduction of injuries and an increase in your performance.

Sample Dynamic Warm-Up Routine (movement based activities):

*Perform each activity for 15-30 seconds while working on a large controlled ROM (range of motion) and repeat the entire circuit for two to three complete rounds.

- Walking High Knees
- Jumping Jacks
- Squats
- Windmills
- Side Lunges
- Reverse Lunge with Spinal Rotation
- Leg Swings (forward and backward)
- Butt Kicks (heels to glutes)
- Arm Swings (forward)
- Arm Swings (backward)
- Cross-Body Arm Swings

STEP #2: RESISTANCE EXERCISE INTERVAL WORKOUT

We'll use two primary workout formats to derive your desired results. The first will be a repetition- based workout. All exercises will require the performance of a specific number of repetitions. The second format will be time-based. All exercises will be performed for a specific time period.

Repetition Based Interval Workouts

Example #1: Bodyweight Only: 6 to 10 Rounds (15-30 minutes)
10 Reaching Jump Squats
10 Wide Push-Ups
10 Jumping Lunges
10 Lying Jackknives
Rest 30 seconds and repeat

Example #2: Bodyweight and Dumbbells: 6 to 10 Rounds (15-30 minutes)
20 Tuck Jumps
10 Dumbbell Alternating Plank Rows
20 Mountain Climbers
10 Dumbbell Swings
20 Lateral Cone Jumps
10 Dumbbell Squats to Overhead Press
Rest 60 seconds and repeat

Example #3: Bodyweight, Dumbbells and a Chair, Box or Step: 3 to 8 Rounds (15-30 minutes)
10 Dumbbell Alternating Overhead Presses
10 Reverse Plank - Alternating Knees to Chin
10 Dumbbell Single Leg RDL's
Rest 30 seconds
10 Dumbbell Squats
10 Plank Salutes
10 Dumbbell Step-Ups
Rest 60 seconds and repeat

Example #4: Bodyweight, Dumbbells and Jump Rope: 3 to 8 Rounds (15-30 minutes)
10 Dumbbell Curl and Squat
10 Burpees
50 Jump Rope Revolutions
Rest 30 seconds
10 Dumbbell Bent Over Rows
10 Close-Grip Push-Ups
50 Jump Rope Revolutions
Rest 60 seconds and repeat

Time Based Interval Workouts

Example #1: Bodyweight Only: 30 second effort – zero rest – 5 to 10 Rounds (17-35 minutes)
Squat Thrust
Plank Hold
Split Squat (each leg)
Push-Up (feet elevated)
Rest 30 seconds and repeat

Example #2: Bodyweight and Dumbbells: 20 second effort – 10 second rest – 4 to 8 Rounds (16-32 minutes)
Jumping Jacks
Dumbbell Alternating Bent Over Row
High Knees
Dumbbell Push-Up (hands on db's)
Pull-Ups or Inverted Rows
Dumbbell Jump Squats
Rest 60 seconds and repeat

Example #3: Bodyweight, Dumbbells and a Chair, Box or Step: 45 second effort – 15 second rest
– 3 to 6 Rounds (18-36 minutes)
Dumbbell Sumo Squats
Plank Rows
Dumbbell Step-Ups
Chair Dips
Dumbbell Walking Lunges
Rest 60 seconds and repeat

Example #4: Bodyweight, Dumbbells and Cone: 60 second effort – 30 second rest
– 2 to 3 Rounds (20-30 minutes)
Dumbbell Clean & Press
Plank (feet elevated)
Dumbbell RDL
Lying Superman X-Up
Dumbbell Lying Chest Press
Lateral Cone Jumps
Rest 90 seconds and repeat

STEP #3: STATIC STRETCHING COOL DOWN

Use this time to allow your muscles to regain their range of motion, your heart rate to gradually come down to a resting level, help reduce post exercise soreness and allow your body to start the recovery process. You'll accomplish this by spending your cool down time performing a series of static stretches.

Hold each stretch for approximately 10 seconds in a static stretched position. Incorporate as many stretches as possible so you cover all your major muscle groups and joints. Examples of muscle groups you should be stretching include:

Hamstrings
Hips
Quadriceps
Calves
Low Back
Chest
Upper Back
Shoulders

YOUR DESIRED RESULTS

Bringing your body to the level of fitness and leanness you desire requires a plan and consistency. What I've outlined for you are the three steps you'll need to take when structuring an effective fat loss exercise program. It's up to you to grasp these simple steps and apply them. You can be certain that if you follow these steps, you'll be well on your way to the physique you desire, with a metabolism primed for maximum fat loss results in minimum time.

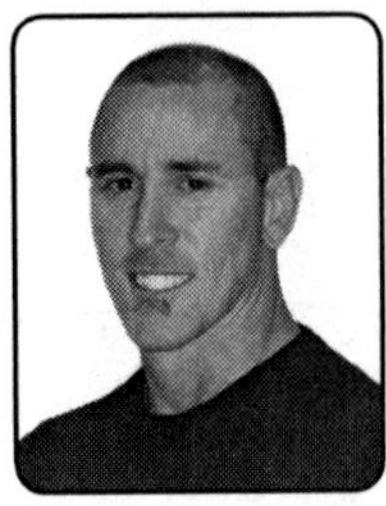

ABOUT ERIC

Eric Gelder is the owner of Body Envy Fitness for Women and is considered Arizona's #1 Fat Loss Expert for Women. He created Body Envy Fitness for the sole purpose of motivating, encouraging and training women to reach their full fitness and fat loss potential in the quickest ways possible.

Eric brings over 16 years of personal training, fitness training management, nutritional consulting and group training experience to Body Envy Fitness. He's also been a contributing writer for the fitness trade publication *Club Success* and has been certified by several national fitness associations – including certifications from ISSA, IFPA and ACE.

Having well over 20,000 documented training sessions with clients under his belt, he has developed his own unique fitness training approach that works, based on real world experience with actual clients. His Body Envy Fitness Training System is highly touted by Arizona women for achieving rapid fat loss results by using simple, effective, proven training and nutritional techniques.

Having spent well over a decade coaching, Eric has successfully integrated his wealth of fitness knowledge into a highly motivating atmosphere, so that clients at Body Envy Fitness can achieve their own dramatic fat loss and fitness results.

As a fitness coach , it is Eric's mission to make fitness a fun, motivating, results-producing activity for women – so that they can achieve all their desired goals – and to support them in developing a lifestyle of health and fitness.

www.EricGelder.com
www.BodyEnvyFitness.com
Contact Eric at 480-686-ENVY (3689)

CHAPTER 20

RENAISSANCE EXERCISE

BY JOSHUA TRENTINE

The historical Renaissance era that occurred in the 14th, 15th, and 16th centuries was not really an awakening as much as it was a RE-awakening of ideas and concepts almost 2000 years old.

Many do not realize that 2,500 years ago, technology was very close to achieving many of the conveniences of modern day, and that this flourishing era was sidetracked by a period of nearly 1000 years of backward thinking called the Dark Ages.

The Dark Ages was a period of economic and cultural deterioration that succeeded in slowing any technical progress and perpetuated man's fears of darkness and the unknown. Barbaric and irrational ideas would gain further power as laws and measures designed to control societies and obliterate free-thinking and opposition.

Similarly, the Dark Age of exercise is characterized by irrational ideas concerning human performance, most notably by so-called *Aerobics Philosophy*. The classical term for *Aerobics* is *steady state* activity. This is any activity that can be carried on *ad infinitum,* – like walking, running, or swimming. This focus on long duration/low-intensity activity represents a myopic failure to consider the entirety of the spectrum of total fitness and physiologic functioning, and thus, a critical example of backward thinking. The activities that we've been told to perform as exercise over the past five decades may be fun and they may provide psychological benefits, but they will not provide sufficient stimulus for continued improvement of the human body. Furthermore, there is a progressively higher and higher risk of physical injury as frequency of activity rises, and as subjects become more intent on achieving their goals. Since these activities never produce the kinds of physique improvements sought out in the first place, they will eventually become psychologically damaging as well, and so begins an endless cycle of guilt, depression, and pain.

Ironically, valid and rational exercise practice and philosophy was making steady progress in ideas up until about 1920. Until then, an emphasis on exercising the skeletal musculature led the way of science and medicine. But various factors including the Great Depression, both world wars, an influenza epidemic and the deaths of many progressive exercise scientists, led the world back to a Dark Age of exercise.

Today's Renaissance Exercise methods are based on stimulating the skeletal muscular system by way of strength-building activity. All reasonable expectations from exercise are accessed through this window by and through strengthening the skeletal muscles. These expectations include improvements in bone density, vascular efficiency, metabolic efficiency, joint stability, muscular strength and cosmetics. Aerobics undermines the necessary process to stimulate strengthening, promotes injuries, and thwarts the body's ability to adapt to the stimulation were it to occur.

It is important for all of us to realize several facts:

- The center of metabolism in the body is the skeletal musculature. Collectively, it possesses the greatest vascularity, the greatest concentration of mitochondria, and the greatest peripheral nerve supply. It is the site of a majority of chemical reactions and heat production.
- Although the heart is a muscle, it is involuntary. It is optimally accessed with exercise only by meaningful muscular (skeletal/volitional) loading. The very nature of steady state (Aerobics) is to avoid meaningful muscular loading by burdening the

bones, so that the muscles are spared to permit endurance and thus avoid exercise.

- *Cardio* makes about as much sense as cutting your heart out of your chest and putting it on an exercise machine.

The key to exercise is strength training. The irrational focus on low intensity, high volume exercise is outdated.

Aerobics represents the Dark Ages of Exercise. Strength Training is the Exercise Renaissance. Do not expect the authorities of the old philosophy to be able to advise you on the principles of the new.

RENAISSANCE METHODS

How much exercise is required for the best results, and how frequently should it be repeated?

This topic is perhaps the most misunderstood issue in the field of exercise today. In most cases, we run into the practice of overworking as opposed to proper training. An attitude of "if some exercise is good, then more must be better" is the most popular mistake. However, many inferior programs emphasize quantity before quality, which is an even more substantial error.

The amount of exercise performed is not the primary determinant for change when creating an exercise program. Many people train twenty or more hours per week without producing the desired results. With Renaissance methods, the minimum requirements are twenty minutes, once a week, although most people get the greatest benefit from training twice a week for 20 minutes of INTENSE training. Under no circumstances should a person train more than three times per week with high intensity efforts. As you grow stronger, your session frequency may be reduced, leaving you even more time for the other stuff in life.

In an hour or less per week with Renaissance methods, much greater results can be achieved, due to a program's focus on **intensity of effort** over total volume of exercise. **Intensity of effort** is the trigger.

"Did you hear that?" ...*INTENSITY OF EFFORT* IS THE TRIGGER!

Here's a little example to help you understand the next concepts. Remember learning math? Addition was first, and it was hard in the beginning. But you practiced a lot, and you learned it. When it came time to learn division, man, was it hard! You had to try to learn it. I'm getting off subject, but my point is, you wouldn't have done a lot of addition, which had become easy for you, in order to get better at division, would you? Even a little bit of practice at that difficult division would get you better results than tons of easy addition. It's similar in exercise. Doing a large amount of an easy chore won't get you anything but a way to pass a lot of time. However, trying your hardest for a small amount of time will bring you better results than you'd ever expected.

In regards to intensity of effort, it is literally impossible to overwork. With most exercise programs, the amount of exercise is often confused with intensity of effort, resulting in a large volume of exercise at minimal efforts.

Trainees need to be skilled in noticing the signs of overtraining, enabling them to prescribe the ideal amount of exercise to produce the best results. This can easily be compared to the proper dosage of medication – too much can be toxic, too little will not produce the desired effect. Exercise in excess can be toxic to the body, resulting in losses of muscle mass, decreases in strength and stamina, susceptibility to illness, insomnia, elevated resting heart rate, and lack of mental focus.

We use brief, high-intensity sessions of exercise with Renaissance methods, using exercise movements that give us the most 'bang for our buck.' Generally, we use what are called compound exercises – exercises that involve several major muscle groups in one movement, so that we can create maximum stimulus without using up our limited resources of energy and motivation. A new subject may start an exercise program in which we simply use three to five compound movements taken to true muscular failure.

If the proper selection of exercise is made, then only a few movements are required to achieve the ultimate level of physical adaptation – "Super body." In the vast majority of cases, the best results will be achieved by using 4 to 7 exercises.

There are some exercises that are generally better than others. These movements will be employed anywhere from one to a maximum of three times per week, and will be challenging to the point of true muscular failure. If performed properly, too much of this type of exercise can quickly lead to a condition of overtraining, which could reverse the results we're trying to produce if taken to an extreme.

In the Renaissance methods program, results will be produced in direct proportion to the intensity of effort. So since you train to get your results, you can probably guess that Renaissance-type exercise is brutally hard work and it must be to produce, and this can be the safest exercise modality. I often warn potential clients who are invited to observe a session that their friend or loved one is not in any pain or danger. Still, I'll usually look over and see the spectator's eyes bulging in fear, as they watch the client's entire body shaking and their breathing extremely labored, as they give their most intense effort. The potential client may begin to doubt that such effort is even possible, or if they do accept the level of effort, they're unwilling to try it. For these reasons, Renaissance methods must be done with a Zen-like focus, which many subjects have described as a meditative or trance state. The trainee's ability to take the body to a place it hasn't been before is the difference between the programs that were never good enough and results beyond your own expectations. You must constantly try to do the momentarily impossible!

There are so many factors involved in exercising properly. To achieve the best results, the ordinary person needs some assistance. A little help to keep them motivated, a little help to keep them at a proper pace of progression, and someone to make sure the exercise is done properly – a qualified instructor will be the difference between status-quo and progress.

One of the key factors in the proven effectiveness of the Renaissance Exercise is the speed of repetitions; here's another little example to help illustrate the importance of the speed of repetitions. Alright, the elevator is broken; you have to take the stairs…up ten flights. You start out at your normal pace then your legs start burning, so you start running. There, that's easier. Then you run out of breath, so you start taking the stairs much slower than you started…we're talking toddler slow. Too slow…you're not getting anywhere. You probably look ridiculous… too fast…while momentum helps take some of the burden off of you, you won't last long at that pace. You could lose control, and you might arrive at your destination sweaty. Find the perfect medium between one step at a time and *Rocky*-style trot, and you'll have the best results. No sweat and you worked those legs a bit.

Too slow a movement is unlikely to bring any desirable results, as the muscles are barely being worked. Too fast a movement relies on momentum, and is also unlikely to bring positive results. Also, exercising at high levels of speed is very difficult to maintain, and can lead to injury…not only is it difficult to judge proper form at high speeds, it's nearly impossible to correct and detect errors. The analogy above is not to be taken as exercise advice, it's just an analogy, the point is we want you to exercise in such a way that puts maximum tension on your muscles, that removes momentum and that, in turn, removes any opportunity to hurt yourself yet radically attenuates your gains.

At Renaissance methods, you can expect most repetitions to take 16-20 seconds. Half of the time used on the positive movement (getting where you need to be) and half for the negative movement (getting back where you started). This optimum speed allows for your trainer to assess your form, improves focus and concentration, causes you to rely on your own strength instead of momentum, and safely gives your muscles the ultimate workout. And you can't cheat!

So, you might be a little overwhelmed at this point - dare I say an overload (btw, overloading muscles is the most fundamental tenet in exercise physiology) of information contradictory to everything you think you know about exercise? At this point, it's time to remember three little nuggets of wisdom:

Let's review:

1. How often you exercise (frequency) is NOT the key to getting successful results from exercise. Intensity is.

2. A small amount of intense exercise is far better than a large amount of easy exercise. (Remember the division vs. addition example)

3. It is crucial to perform movements at the optimum speed in order to realize the most intense effort, and produce the best results.

It's a lot to absorb, and we're just getting started. It's most important to produce intense effort at all times, monitor your progress, and so much more.

So... you've given Renaissance methods a try; ...you've learned to give your most intense effort ...you've learned to use the machines properly; ...you're even getting the hang of the proper speed of motion. It only gets easier now, right?

NO!! DON'T BELIEVE EVERYTHING YOU THINK IS CORRECT!

It's not going to get easier. Not the way you think, anyway. You will know what you're doing, but the effort given will always be your greatest. You will always have to try to improve upon what you did before, ...more time doing a movement (time under load), additional weight, new exercises, a new sequence. Any and all of these changes will be made so that no workout will ever be exactly the same ...a little thing known as progress.

As you continue with the program, you'll start to notice an increase in your strength and endurance – you'll be working as hard as when you began the program, but doing more than ever (be it more time under load, increased weight, whatever).

The great variety provided by the Renaissance methods program will force your body to adapt in ways you've never seen.

- Increased Strength
- Greater Endurance
- Increased calorie burning, even while doing nothing
- Reduction in body fat
- Improved cardiovascular health
- More energy
- General sense of well-being

Your muscles are getting stronger! You're gaining muscle! You might be getting tighter where you once jiggled! Holy smokes, this Renaissance stuff feels like its working! There are more benefits to exercise than just strength, endurance, and improved appearance. You'll notice you just start feeling better in general. You'll notice that increased energy and a more positive outlook leave you able to get more out of your days, as busy as they already are. You'll jump over life's little hurdles a bit faster, too…carrying groceries, climbing the stairs; everything will just start to come a bit easier.

It's a challenge to keep that progress going. You might expect to plateau, that dreaded word in exercise and diet books worldwide. Many exercise programs are guilty of abandonment on the plateau …getting a subject near their goal, then providing no plan of action to improve upon, or at least maintain the desired level of fitness. Don't you just hate that?

A few tips, often overlooked, that can go a long way:

TRAINING ENVIRONMENT

#1 – "IT'S COLD IN HERE!"

Ideally a facility's temperature should always hover between 61 and 65 degrees Fahrenheit, with strategically-placed oscillating fans. Think of your body as an automobile for a moment. Your muscles are the motors. As they work hard giving all of that intense effort, they give off heat, raising the needle on your heat gauge.

Much like your car is less likely to overheat in winter than in summer, our bodies are better served by exercise in cooler environments. The heat escapes into the air!

#2 – "WHERE'S THE MUSIC?"

Ideal facilities are devoid of any distractions. There are no mirrors, televisions, or loud music to interrupt the subject's concentration. You came to the gym to exercise, not to dance, flirt, or watch the latest sports highlights.

Remember, you won't be spending endless time on a treadmill, needing music to keep you motivated. You'll be moving from machine to machine after three minutes or less… Watching yourself in a mirror is an unnecessary distraction.

Did we mention you won't sweat??? Sweating is your body's evaporative cooling mechanism; it means you are overheating, NOT that you're getting a good workout.

#3 – TAKE A BREAK

With Renaissance methods, your workouts will be challenging and intense, to the point of momentary muscular failure. At this level, it is crucial to avoid overtraining. The body needs to rest in order to continue to progress. It is recommended that you allow at least two days between sessions. Three is usually better. Exercise is, at its very core, damaging your muscles. Sounds scary, doesn't it? In proper doses, high-intensity exercise is just the kind of damage your body needs. During the recovery period, your muscles heal, and adjust to their recent efforts. Performing such intense exercise again too soon will restrict any desired results. There will be times when a subject just needs a break from training, …illness, injury, vacation, family or work obligations, or rarely, just a psychological rut.

These layoffs are permitted, and layoffs have their benefits. When you come back, you'll have a greater enthusiasm, and any losses in strength will be easily regained.

Intensity- important!
Frequency- not as important!
Speed- crucial to quality!
Progression- always grow!
Equipment- essential!
Environment- distraction-free is best!
Recovery- take a break!

There's one more crucial factor to the success of an exercise program. In fact it may be the most important factor:

CONFIDENCE

If you say you can't do something, you'll usually prove yourself right. However, the power of intention works for good, as well. They didn't teach "if you believe it, you can achieve it" in high school for nothing.

When it comes to the human body, there are basic biological laws that exist. If the body is momentarily exposed to stress, a threat, something above and beyond what it is used to (by definition this is called *Overload*), then there will be a cascade of biological events that occur as the body synthesizes a response. No amount of low-level non-specific activity can elicit this response. The Renaissance exerciser should be aware that a specific process exists and that the body is governed by biological laws.

Once we are aware of the process, and we follow with sufficient *Overload,* we can rest at ease that we have done everything in our power to bring our body to its genetic potential ... and we can do so in a minimum amount of time in order to allow for other pursuits, and become a true Renaissance man or woman.

LET THE RENASSIANCE BEGIN!

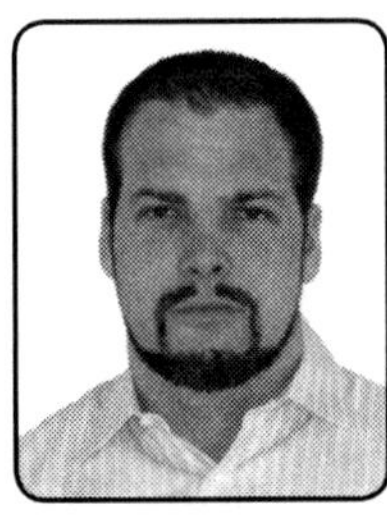

ABOUT JOSH

Joshua Trentine is the founder of Renaissance Exercise, an online authority in the High Intensity Strength Training industry, and Overload Fitness, one of the country's premier one-on-one personal training facilities with two locations in the greater Cleveland, Ohio area and a third facility in Altamonte Springs, Florida.

Joshua has always been fascinated by physical culture, starting in his early teens. It was this fascination that has given him a broad spectrum of knowledge in the health and fitness industry. Joshua has an extensive background in physical therapy and nutrition and fitness. He has used his extensive knowledge to achieve the highest level (Professional) in the natural drug-free body building arena. Joshua has used his expertise and personal experience to help hundreds of clients achieve their health and fitness goals – in minimal time spent away from their daily lives.

Joshua has been featured on Super Human Radio, ESPN Radio, CBS Radio, That's Life with Robin Swoboda, FOX 8 News, The Cleveland Plain Dealer and countless other on-line forums and discussion groups. Joshua also does public speaking and has contributed to several publications throughout his career. He is also a well respected and sought after authority in the High-Intensity community.

Meet him at www.overloadfitness.com and www.renaissanceexercise.com.

CHAPTER 21

ESSENTIAL GROUND RULES FOR EFFECTIVE TEN-MINUTE WORKOUTS

BY ROMMEL ACDA

In my fitness consulting business, I have the opportunity to consult with people from all walks of life about their health and fitness goals. These goals range from losing stubborn body fat, gaining muscle, getting stronger, to putting together a nutrition program that fits into their busy lifestyle, or simply a plan to stay in shape all year round. Regardless of their goals there seems to be one common fitness culprit – TIME.

Life doesn't play fair for many of us, and because of that TIME has become the number one challenge in our quest to stay in shape. I've definitely had my fair share of struggles with time:

a. Too much to do
b. No time for a workout and
c. Too busy to cook today so I'm going through the drive-thru

You see, a couple years ago I woke up feeling out-of-shape, exhausted, and embarrassed with the physique I saw in the mirror. I think a lot of people can relate. However, my particular problem was that I am a fitness professional with 10 years of experience.

Nine months prior to this moment, I had embarked on an opportunity that I knew was going to change my life completely. I decided to quit my full-time position as a personal trainer at a very high-end athletic club, and start my own fitness consulting company.

I didn't want to be tied down to a "job" anymore, and felt that I needed more "freedom of expression" with my career, and the only way for that to happen was to go independent.

Fast forward nine months and I was making good money, but I was highly stressed from having to juggle three roles - new business owner, personal trainer, and husband. I had a hard time balancing career and family responsibilities, along with other typical life demands.

A once typical day for me:

- 4:00 am Wake up, go to work, and instruct a fitness boot camp
- 7:00 am Eat "second" breakfast
- 8:00 am Answer emails
- 9:00 am Setup a newsletter or blog
- 10:00 am Snack time :)
- 11:00 am More training clients
- 12:00 pm Eat lunch, then errands
- 2:00 pm Workout...oh wait, need to deal with a misunderstanding between two of my staff members :(
- 3:00 pm Snack, then maybe a workout...oops, forgot to send out an email
- 4:00 pm Instruct fitness boot camps
- 6:00 pm Workout...crap! Never mind, the wife needs me to run to the grocery store, guess I'll get a quick workout at home instead
- 7:00 pm Get home, mentally exhausted, make excuse that I'll just get my workout in tomorrow, because now I'm starving as well, and simply want to unwind at this point

I had never experienced this type of stress before, and I found myself making the same excuses my clients would give me: "I just don't have the time to fit in a workout!"

What???

I am a fitness professional and I couldn't even practice what I preach because I allowed my mindset to be compromised from all the stress. Epic Fail!

So, as I looked at myself in the mirror again, I simply said, "Stop it, you're better than this! Now go fix it because you know exactly how to fix it!"

I did, in fact, know how to fix it. Just a few years before this I was designing short and effective ten minute workouts for my extremely busy clients. Clients who were CEO's, General Managers, small business owners, stay-at-home moms - you name that busy person, and I guarantee you I've trained them.

I came up with a solution to help them not just get back into shape, but to stay in shape at home, on lunch hour at work, or on travels. So why wasn't I using this very solution I created?

Because I was still of the mindset that for my own personal workouts and fitness goals, these short workouts were not appropriate. I had to take a good look at all that I had designed. As I dissected the information, I had some "a-ha!" moments that there were components that would absolutely work for me.

But while re-discovering these components, I also determined that there were certain shortcomings that needed to be addressed, and that in order to be effective, these 10-minute workouts needed to meet the following criteria:

1. They had to be simple, yet fun.
2. They needed to be able to be performed anywhere - at home, the gym, hotel room, or outdoors - with little to no equipment.
3. They needed to be challenging enough in the short amount of time in order to make a difference to the body.
4. They needed to be strategic in program design in order to

avoid plateaus and allow consistent progress.

5. They needed to have periodic "fitness challenges" as a means to test and challenge fitness levels.

After creating my first 12 weeks of workouts, I started testing them out on myself. I expected to confirm that my workouts were simply a solution for staying in shape and maintaining body strength. But within just a few short weeks I noticed a dramatic change in conditioning, strength, and body fat reduction!

I mentioned these findings to a client and his response was, "Bulls**t"! It will never work!" ... and then he accused me of being a low rate infomercial. Needless to say, he 'pissed me off', so I went to work into more research as to why these methods were working. In addition, I recruited a few other clients with busy schedules to further demonstrate these short workouts produced results.

Briony was a single mom who only had a short window of time to exercise between work and cooking dinner for her son. Dave was a CEO and husband whose busy schedule allowed him no time to go to the gym. Using my 10-minute workouts, Briony lost her post-pregnancy weight and got back to her bikini-ready body. Dave regained his core fitness and enjoyed pain-free road cycling and skiing for the first time in years.

My clients definitely appreciated that my workouts took so little time out of their days. What they didn't know was that these short workouts were designed with key principles in mind that made them highly effective.

So based on my findings, here are:

THE 5 ESSENTIAL PRINCIPLES FOR EFFECTIVE 10-MINUTE WORKOUTS

1. Basic total body exercises should be emphasized with a fusion of core and specialty exercises to keep it interesting and fun.

2. To maintain strength, the "work set" needs to last 20-30 seconds; and to maintain endurance and conditioning, the "work set" needs to last between 45-60 seconds.

3. For strength, choose a resistance that is challenging for a set of 5 reps, and for muscular endurance choose a resistance that is challenging for a set of 10 reps.

4. Repetition speed needs to be performed as quickly as possible, provided form is not compromised. If form is compromised the set needs to be terminated.

5. Rest-to-work ratio needs to be equal for strength gains, but cut rest in half if endurance and conditioning is desired.

If designed to uphold these principles, a 10-minute workout can yield amazing results. My clients, although skeptical at first, are a walking testament to that.

Okay, so you're ready for the workouts, right? Wrong!

What I also learned through this whole process is that before diving into any fitness program, *you must do 3 things to set yourself up for success:*

1. SIMPLIFY YOUR FITNESS GOALS

Simplify your fitness goals to 1-2 items. Why? Because, too many goals on your list will set you up for failure by becoming overbearing as you lose motivation.

So how do you avoid losing the spark? In setting your goals, you must ask yourself these important questions:

Why is this important to me?

What action steps am I willing to do, and sacrifices am I willing to make?

What things am I NOT willing to do?

How will finally achieving my goal make me feel?
...and what do I gain?

When you ask yourself these questions you now add true substance, and create a bigger "Why". The "Why" is what will ultimately help you maintain that motivational spark.

Lastly, **WRITE IT DOWN!** Write down your goals and the answers to the questions above. Keep it somewhere easily accessible and turn to it whenever you need to spark things up again.

2. CREATE YOUR PLAN AND WORK IT WITH PASSION

So you've set your goals. Now put together a plan of action with all the support structures you feel you need in order to successfully navigate this plan. Set a realistic time frame to achieve your goals, figure out all the possible roadblocks you'll run into, THEN create the weekly structure that you know will work in your lifestyle to overcome these obstacles. Once this is created, you've won half the battle, because this plan will help maintain the discipline to keep your goals in your sights.

Things to consider in creating your structure:

- Healthy, supportive foods that you enjoy and are easy to incorporate into your lifestyle (Remember, supportive nutrition will account for 80% of your goal)
- Set up a consistent time to get your workouts in
- Get the support you need from family and friends, put your goals out there, heck more than likely one of them will ask to join you on your journey
- Schedule a reward every 3 weeks, such as a massage, or night out with a loved one or friends. This helps keep you sane and looking forward to showing off your progress - (trust me, they'll notice)
- Create a vision/motivation board full of inspiring pictures and quotes, and hang it where you'll see it

3. GET OVER IT!

Every week I hear clients telling me every "good story" in their book as to why they're not achieving the results they want. They point fingers elsewhere when they should be pointing at themselves.

Only you can push yourself harder in a workout, only you can put non-nutritious food in your mouth, and only you can control your time to dedicate to your fitness plan and achieve the results you're looking for.

As a fitness professional, I'm here to help motivate you and to provide you with the tools and the "map" to your fitness goals, but I'm not the one to drive you there. It's not my role or place.

Just get rid of the excuses, and get done what needs to be done. Take small steps if needed, but just understand that every small step achieved is a victory not a challenge.

At least you took action, and that's better than 90% of the individuals out there. Take inspired action, and before you know it you've achieved the results you've been looking for.

Now that you've simplified and written down your goals, created your action plan, and gotten over your boring excuses, you're ready to get going! In the attached Addendum are two sample routines to get you started. Again, simple yet effective. Please remember to warm-up properly before partaking in any of these workouts. Have fun!

ADDENDUM

Workout 1: equipment needed – fitness bands

Protocol (timed sets): perform each exercise in a circuit for 30 seconds of work time, rest 10 seconds between exercises, complete 4 rounds.

1. Squat to Row
2. Standing Band Plank into Band Twists (twist from left to right)
3. Forward Lunge to Chest Press
4. Standing Band Plank into Band Twists (twist from right to left)

Workout 2: equipment needed – dumbbells

Protocol (timed sets): Option 1 - perform each exercise for 30 seconds, rest 10 seconds, complete 3 rounds; Option 2 - perform each exercise for 40 seconds, rest 10 seconds, complete 2 rounds; perform as a circuit just like Workout #1.

1. Reverse Lunge to Shoulder Press
2. Plank Row (each side)
3. Dumbbell Get-Ups (each side)

** Tip: Attempt this without a dumbbell first. If you are unable to maintain vertical arm position, then you must first build-up your core strength and stability before you can start to add dumbbell resistance.

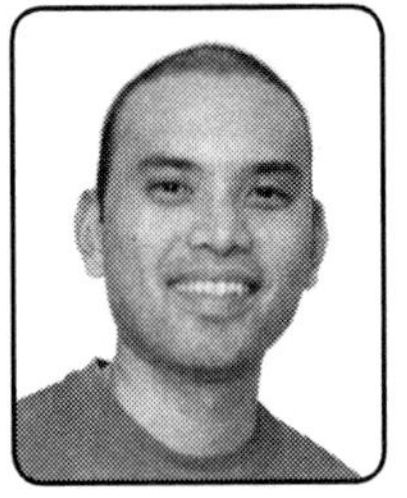

ABOUT ROMMEL

Rommel Acda is a fitness professional with 12 years of experience in the industry. He is a Certified Strength and Conditioning Specialist (CSCS), and co-owner of Element 5 Fitness Training Center in Kirkland, Washington.

Rommel built his fitness business by helping hundreds of busy clients – from top business executives to real estate agents and busy moms – achieve amazing shape and regain their health and their bodies. His latest fitness system, "Fit In A Hurry", is a culmination of his 'in-the-trenches' work with his busy clientele, as well as his juggling of a very busy schedule running his business and being a new father.

By identifying what is crucial for a ten-minute workout, Rommel is able to mesh specific fitness protocols to maximize his clients' results in minimum time.

To learn more about Rommel Acda, and how you can receive free workouts, special reports, and other invaluable fitness and fat loss information for the busy person, visit: www.fitinahurry.com/blog. If you live in the Greater Seattle/Eastside area of Washington State and would like to work with Rommel one-on-one, please visit: www.element5fitness.com or call 425-823-4400 or Toll-Free 1-877-823-4939 to schedule a free consultation.

CHAPTER 22

THE TOP FIVE SECRETS TO HAVING A DANCER'S BODY

– IN 45 MIN. OR LESS PER DAY!

BY KRISTEN NOLAN

With the rise in popularity of shows like "So You Think You Can Dance" and "Dancing with the Stars", getting that perfect dancer's body has become something that more and more people desire. Dancers have the long, lean and toned look that every woman wants. Their bodies are defined and not bulky and 'butch'. Most people I talk to think that it would be impossible for them to achieve a dancer's body without actually being a professional dancer, which is certainly not true at all. In fact, before I became a personal trainer and learned the top five secrets to getting that toned "dancer look," I was a part-time salsa dancer in my mid-20s and certainly didn't have the body of one! Before that, I had been dancing my entire life – ballet, jazz, tap, salsa, you name it. When I was a teenager things seemed to stay in place on my body, no jiggly belly, thighs or arms! I ate what I wanted, and all I had to do was dance. Life was good.

Then, I got an office job and became less active – only going to dance practice twice a week and visiting the vending machines at work every time I got a sweet craving. My metabolism slowed down and I started gaining weight.

At this point, I didn't realize why my body was changing so drastically. I felt at a loss, how could something I had been doing my entire life stop working for me? I felt uncomfortable when I had to get on a stage and wear flashy costumes or dress up in skirts and tight tops to go dancing with my friends. I desperately wanted my teenage-dancer body back. But when I decided to start trying to change my life and get my dancer-look back, I didn't know where to start…

I began months of experimentation. No carbs, no fat, low fat, protein only, no fruit, tons of ab crunches, hours of 'cardio' on the elliptical staying in the "fat burning zone" – what a waste! And without having a proper fitness background at the time, I had no clue what the right answer was to get fast results. Everything I would read had conflicting and confusing information.

Finally, I hooked up with excellent fitness coaches. They helped me toss all those crazy ideas out the window and find a nutrition and exercise solution that worked for me.

After applying all the information I learned, I ended up getting my lean and toned body back, and in my opinion, even better than it was when I was younger! This inspired me to help other people achieve the same results I did. I got my National Academy of Sports Medicine Personal Training license and went to work, sharing all the information I could with my clients – on how to achieve that nice, lean and toned "dancer" look with their bodies. This is what I will share with you all today!

Here are the top 5 secrets I applied to Achieve a Fit Dancer's Body:

1. I got my diet on track
2. I started cardiovascular Interval Training
3. Trained my core
4. Learned strength training and stretching techniques to tone and elongate my muscles
5. Developed a Weekly Fitness Plan and remained consistent with my efforts

NOW TO YOU! HERE ARE THE DETAILS:—

SECRET #1
GETTING YOUR DIET ON TRACK

When I was looking to get my dancer body back, one of the biggest lessons I learned was that my diet had played a major role in my weight gain. No matter how hard I exercised, that fat would not fall off without getting my diet back on track. There are 4 steps to getting this right:

STEP 1 – FOOD JOURNALING

Fit dancers are very strict about what they put in their mouth because they want to look good in their costumes and feel lighter during their performances. So, to get the lean figure you desire you must first learn how you can change your eating habits to reduce your waist size and feel more energized. Food journals are an amazing tool to help you determine if you are eating the correct balance of healthy proteins, carbs and fats per day.

Food journals can be done fast, in about 5 min. a day! The goal is to record when you eat, what you eat and drink, approximate portion of food and number of calories consumed. Last, note how you are feeling, especially if you are eating a reduced number of calories for weight loss. This will allow you to remember how good you feel when you eat certain foods, and assess what you can be doing to get better results.

STEP 2 – EAT BALANCED MEALS EVERY 3-4 HOURS, OR 4-5 SMALL MEALS A DAY.

Dancers do this so their bodies remain energized during their practices and their heads stay focused on their choreography and not the fact that they are hungry.

When I initially tell clients this, the first thing they say to me is "I don't have time." The good news is that this doesn't have to take much time at all. The trick to eating every 3-4 hours is to plan, shop and prepare your meals before your hectic week begins. For me, the best day to do this is Sunday. "Each meal should consist of a protein (lean meat, eggs, fish, high quality protein powder), non-starchy carbohydrates (TONS of leafy, crunchy vegetables, think colors), and about 2 thumb sizes of healthy fat (coconut oil, walnuts, almonds, chia seeds, flax seeds olive oil, avocado). Minimize your starchy and heavier carbohydrates. When you do eat them, try to select from whole grains such as quinoa, buckwheat and millet, legumes, and sweet potatoes. Maybe try going a day or 2 without them. You will feel lighter! This combination helps the nutrients release slowly into your system to keep you satisfied and focused. Once you build a habit of doing this, it becomes second nature. Here are some examples of healthy food combinations that I eat every week:

Breakfast:

– 2 eggs with 3 cups of mixed greens (spinach, arugula, kale)

Lunch/Dinner

– Grilled Chicken on top of a large mixed greens salad with red peppers, mushrooms, seeds and olive oil
– Salmon and sauteed spinach, onions and garlic
– Lean Steak with mixed grilled vegetables

Healthy Snacks:

– Piece of fruit and raw nuts
– 1/2 Avocado with 2 slices lean turkey
– Celery and almond butter
– Scoop of protein powder and fresh fruit smoothie

** **Extra Tip** – Remember to load your plate with a ton of non-starchy veggies (mixed greens, kale, chard, peppers, etc) as much as possible. Aim to hit 10 + cups a day! This can be done easily by adding at least 3 cups of veggies to every meal and 1 cup to every snack.

STEP 3 – CONTROL YOUR PORTIONS

Dancers do this to have flat stomachs. You could be eating the cleanest foods in the world, but if you are eating too much your body will be storing the extra food as fat. Calories are calories no matter where they come from. Look at your portions and become aware of when your body is full. Here are 2 indications that your portion size was too large:

- You feel sluggish after a meal (you want to go to sleep) - You do not feel energized from your food.

- Your clothes feel tight – If your pants feel much tighter after you've eaten a meal, your portion was probably too large.

** **Extra Tip** – It is very hard to tell when you are full if you get to your meal starving, don't ever let yourself get too hungry!

STEP 4 – EAT CLEAN FOODS!

Your grocery shopping must be done on the exterior of the grocery store. Shop for foods like veggies, fruits, lean proteins, whole grains, healthy fats, nuts. Read labels, if you cannot pronounce the ingredients on a label, chances are the food is not good for you!

Avoid purchasing foods with white sugars, white flour, sauces, yogurt with sugary mixes, sodas, processed baked goods, most packaged food such as cereals, crackers, and chips. Keeping your diet clean, healthy and well-balanced will reduce your sugar cravings, give you more energy for your day and help you become leaner so you feel better about yourself. And once this happens, you will feel great starting your workout plan!

SECRET #2
CARDIOVASCULAR TRAINING LIKE A DANCER TO LOSE FAT

Now that you have the diet of a dancer, it is time to train like one. The easiest way to start this is by changing your cardio sessions from medium-paced, hour- long sessions to 20-30 min. cardio sessions with intense bursts of energy also known as High Intensity Interval Training or (HITT). Dancers need a 'ton' of stamina to make it through a performance, but they also need to develop the cardiovascular strength to expend energy at the peaks of their shows. Evidently this is also the type of cardiovascular training that burns the most fat and calories overall.

HITT will:

- Build and retain lean muscle mass
- Target metabolically active fat (most visible fat, especially around mid section)

- Burn the most calories overall and increase fat utilization during and after exercise!
- *Interval Training* is so effective that you even burn calories post workout.

The reason more people do not train this way is because it is hard! You really have to give it your all. There is also a huge myth that doing slow cardio and staying in the so-called "fat burning zone" will be most effective for fat loss. Just to put it in perspective, sitting down all day burns calories from fat! My point is that it does not matter where the calories come from when the most effective way to lose fat is to burn the most calories overall.

Here is a great way to start and develop your *Interval Training* regime. Please note that you can use any cardio machine for this method. I like the Treadmill and Stair Climber the best. For this example, I will use the Treadmill:

Start your session with a 5 min. warm up! Then choose one of the following levels and perform 5-10 sets:

- Beginner Level 1 = 1 min. fast run – 3 min. walk or light jog
- Intermediate Level 2 = 1 min. fast run – 2 min. walk or light jog
- Advanced Level 3 = 1 min. fast run – 1 min. walk or light jog

** **Extra tip** – To push this along, play with the timing of your fast-cardio burst. For example, the shorter your fast run is, the harder you can work for this time. If you are only running for 15-30 seconds, you can choose a higher speed on the treadmill than you could if you were running fast for 1 minute.

SECRET #3
TRAIN YOUR CORE LIKE A DANCER

Dancers need strong cores to hold their balance and to keep their movements controlled to appear effortless. They also have incredible postures, which also comes from core strength.

Without getting into too much detail, your core consists of over ten major muscles in the abdomen, back and glutes. The reason I want to emphasize core training is because once you have a good idea of how to stabilize this section, you can move on to the full-body strength and conditioning exercises that will ultimately get you the dancer's body you desire.

To develop excellent core-stabilization and posture, you will want to train the core in it's entirety. Planks are a great place to start. Be sure that your whole spine from the top of your head to your tailbone is in alignment. (You never want your hips to drop below your chest, as it puts loads of pressure on the lower back.) Other core-stabilization exercises include the side plank (for abs, back and glutes), hip press (for glutes and lower back), lat pull down (for latissimus dorsi) and upright row (for upper back and postural muscles).

SECRET #4
STRENGTH TRAINING TO TONE YOUR MUSCLES AND STRETCHING TO ELONGATE MUSCLES

Dancers' bodies have to be strong in order to hold their legs in the air and to execute lifts and tricks with their dance partners by holding their own body weight. To do this well, they must do strength training.

Proper and consistent strength training 3-4 days a week:

(a) reduces body fat
(b) speeds up our metabolism so we burn more calories at rest
(c) builds bone density, and
(d) tones and strengthens the entire body.

I have found that the most effective strength training to lean the body is to perform compound movements one after the other with little rest. This not only trains multiple body parts at a time but also provides a cardio element to your workout. This can only be done safely after you have mastered moving one body part at a time (e.g., core, legs, arms).

Here are some examples of my favorite compound exercises:

- Squat + shoulder press (legs and arms)

- Push up (chest and core)
- Row – biceps and back
- Forward walking lunges with dumbbells – glutes, quads, calves
- Wood chops – core and shoulders
- Deadlifts – glutes, quads, calves, core
- Single leg squats – glutes, quads, calves, core
- Pull Up – core, lats, back

Remember, after all workouts, you will want to stretch and elongate the muscles. Stretching while your muscles are warm allows you to increase your flexibility, avoid getting too sore post-workout, and avoid injury.

SECRET #5
HAVING A PLAN AND REMAINING CONSISTENT

The biggest secret to being successful in this program is that you must develop your weekly plan. Include your nutrition/meal preparation, your strength training and cardiovascular workouts. Then, stick with the plan and remain consistent with your efforts. I've found that through making healthy nutrition choices and prioritizing my workouts, I have been able to reach and maintain the body changes I have worked so hard for. This doesn't mean you can't ever fall off track.

There will be parties, vacations and sometimes life gets in the way! The trick is not to beat yourself up about it. If you do have a day where you fall off-track, cut your losses and get straight back on. It is much easier to get yourself back on track after one day off than after three days off. This is also the way you will develop your nutrition and workout efforts into a habit so these things become second nature.

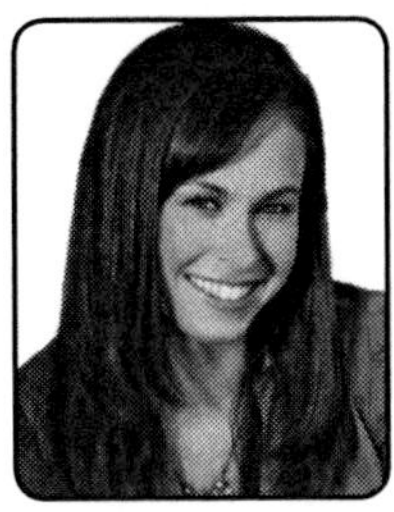

ABOUT KRISTEN

Kristen Nolan is a professional salsa dancer and NASM certified Personal Trainer. She owns a successful Fitness Boot Camp and Personal Training business in San Francisco, CA called "I Luv My Body Fitness." Her company specializes in helping women and men lose fat, lean and tone their bodies, and get healthy.

Kristen started her Personal Training and Salsa Dancing career in her twenties after struggling with her own weight loss battles. Since then she has combined her knowledge from the worlds of fitness and dance to develop her own proven, step-by-step exercise methods to help women and men reach their ideal figures. She also works closely with a partner to integrate nutrition programs and healthy supplementation for weight loss and maintenance to her clients.

Kristen has placed in the top 3 in several World Salsa Dancing Competitions with her Teams Couture Dance Alliance and Salsamania located in the San Francisco Bay Area. These include 1st Place in the San Francisco Salsa Congress 2010, 1st Place in the Semi Final Rounds of the World Latin Cup 2010, 1st place US Salsa Open 2010, 1st Place Roccapulco Salsa Competition 2009, 3rd Place at the ESPN World Salsa Championships in 2006, and 2nd Place in the World Salsa Championships 2005.

To learn more about Kristen Nolan and how you can receive free health and fitness reports from her company, visit: www.iluvmybody.com or call 1-877-359-3633.

CHAPTER 23

THE SECRET TO ULTIMATE FITNESS AND WELLNESS:

TRAIN LIKE AN ATHLETE

BY VAUGHN BETHELL

Have you ever noticed how competitive athletes tend to have the best looking bodies? I'm sure you have. Think of Olympic sprinters, football players, basketball players, soccer players, boxers, mixed martial artists, and the list goes on. The majority of these athletes are pretty muscular, lean, and have the picture-perfect physique or beach body that the 'average Joe' would love to have.

Believe me I know. In the 9 years that I have been training others, it seems like every personal training client comes in with aspirations of having a body like their favorite athlete. Before I go any further on this topic I want you to first consider why exactly you work out. You are working out aren't you?

If weight loss is your main goal then you probably want to ***look*** more like an athlete right?

If getting stronger or running faster is your main goal you probably want to ***perform*** like an athlete…

And if your main goal is to just stay healthy and prevent injury you definitely want to ***train*** like an athlete. Starting to get the picture?

Fortunately for me I got into sports and athletics at an early age. My father played soccer for the Bahamas National Team, so needless to say, he had me on the field as soon as I was old enough. I didn't draw the line at soccer though, while growing up I played baseball, basketball, and football as well. My parents let me try out everything until I was mature enough to make my own decision as to which one I wanted to stick with. I encourage you to do the same with your children, as it will help them embrace sports and specifically an active lifestyle.

I personally chose to pursue soccer. I was a good overall athlete, and probably above average in each sport that I played, compared to those I was competing with, but I was the best in soccer. I stood out from the crowd, and it led to playing at the Division I Collegiate Level and eventually numerous appearances for the Bahamas National Team, which included two World Cup Qualifying stints for Germany 2006 and South Africa 2010. It must run in the family.

It's funny because even though I grew up as an athlete, and had much success in my sport (believe me, it didn't come easy), I always considered my training as part of my athletic career, and that when I finished playing I could leave all of that behind. Old folks (at the time I was 20) don't need to train like this, right?

Boy was I wrong!

In college, I majored in Health and Exercise Science, and in my senior year I started an internship at a one-on-one personal training studio. It was your old-fashioned traditional personal training with wall-to-wall machines and a whole lot of rep counting. Monday: "Back and bi's", Wednesday: "Chest and tris", Friday: legs. You know the routine.

It amazed me how routine everything was, and to me routine is boring! Not just to me, but boring to your body as well. I don't know about you, but when I'm bored I can easily fall asleep. Well, your body is the same way and when it gets into a routine, it might as well be asleep because it's really not benefiting from the program anymore. You should have seen it. The clients at this studio might as well have been paying for a country club membership.

The turning point for me came about 6 months later, by this time I had completed my internship and they had hired me on full time. I went into work one Saturday morning and when I arrived, there was a sign on the door that read, 'We are no longer in business!' Wow, the owner not only didn't bother to tell the clients, but he took off without even telling his trainers! I guess you can't run a successful personal training business if you fail to provide results.

Well, believe it or not, that day turned out to be the best day of my life. It's when I decided that I wanted to work primarily with athletes and I was going to do it on my own. I started training my own clients out of another studio and at local sports fields. In a relatively short period of time, I had built up enough clientele that I opened up my own training facility. That was January 2005.

At the time, the majority of my clients were competitive athletes ranging from the ages of 8 to18, but not long after opening up shop, parents of the athletes I was training started asking me if I would be willing to work with them. They saw what I was doing with their children and the results they were getting, and they said it looked like FUN to them. The medicine balls, the bungee cords, the bands, the big inflatable ball... Without much thought, my response was "Of Course!"

Why not? They liked what they saw and they trusted me. So I began to train these adults the same way as I was training my younger competitive athletes. Why separate them? We're all after the same thing anyway, right?

In just a short period of time after working with these "amateur athletes", something amazing started happening...they saw results faster than they ever thought possible. One client lost 13lbs and 7% body fat in the first six weeks.

Well today, results like that are normal around my facility. In fact, as I sit here writing this, we are starting into 2011, and out of the nearly 200 clients that we are currently working with, more than 75% of them are adult "amateur athletes." Part of that has to do with the fact that we only train serious elite high school, college, and professional athletes now. But whether you're looking to get stronger and faster, or simply lose weight and drop body fat, results speak and the word has gotten out.

So how exactly do athletes train? Well, that is highly dependent on their sport, but one thing I can tell you is that they don't have "back and bi's" or "chest and tri's" days.

Now before I get into how to train like an athlete, there a few things you must embrace first:

I. Change your workouts (no more routine)
   - Changing your workouts will not only change your body, it can change your life

II. Change your mindset (get your mind right)
   - Change your mind about what a workout is supposed to be, and what you need to do in the gym to make it work for you

III. Push beyond your limits
   - Like a great strength coach once told me "Get Comfortable With the Uncomfortable," doing this helps you achieve what seemed impossible

Once you understand these things, you are ready to roll!

So let's get to it! Below are three musts to training like an athlete:

1. DYNAMIC WARM-UP

It is ridiculous the way most people warm up – 5 to 10 minutes on the treadmill or the elliptical to start, a few static stretches here and there, maybe a couple of crunches or something. This "warm-up" is pointless. It doesn't warm your body up properly, which can lead to injuries. And it doesn't prepare your body for the kind of effort you need to put in if you want your workouts to be productive.

A proper warm-up should make you sweat. It fires up your entire neuromuscular system.

In our facility we use a series of mobility exercises, coordination exercises, and conditioning exercises. All you need is about 20-30 feet of floor space. The exercises typically include high knees, butt kicks, A skips, B skips, knee hugs, cradle walks, high kicks, lunge with a twist, side lunges, shuffles, carioca, jump squats, jump lunges, and more. You can see these exercises performed on our website at: www.greenvillepersonaltrainers.com. Once you're used to it, a dynamic warm-up takes between 7 to 10 minutes.

2. FUNCTIONAL TRAINING

I will define functional training or "functional movement training" as training that allows our bodies to function at an optimal level. Athletes train for function to create stronger, more athletic physiques in order to prevent injury and compete in their sport.

Since our bodies function as a whole unit it would also make more sense to train our whole body during each session rather than isolating each muscle group. Muscles don't function in isolation in the real world so why would we train them that way? At our facility we have very few machines because most of them isolate muscle groups. In the case of bodybuilding this is okay because they need repetitive body part training for gaining excessive muscle mass.

However, the rest of us who would rather build a healthier, more athletic looking body should focus on training 'movements' rather than 'muscles'. So unless you are a professional or aspiring bodybuilder, consider yourself an athlete.

Here are seven basic 'functional' movement patterns you should be training:

- ✓ Horizontal pressing movements (e.g. push ups)
- ✓ Horizontal pulling movements (e.g. inverted row)
- ✓ Vertical pulling movements (e.g. pull-ups)
- ✓ Vertical pushing movements (e.g. push presses)
- ✓ Quad dominant exercises (e.g. squats, lunges)
- ✓ Hip dominant exercises (e.g. deadlifts)
- ✓ Rotational/Twisting movements (e.g. med ball throws)

Functional training consists of compound or multi-joint movements generally targeting the large muscle groups, which burn a huge amount of calories, and stimulates metabolism, but also hits the smaller muscle groups as well as the stabilizers and proprioceptors. It's not uncommon for me to hear clients saying that they are "sore in places that they didn't even know that they had!"

3. HIGH INTENSITY WORKOUTS

Gone are the days of spending an hour and a half to two hours in the gym. Training like an athlete means efficient exercise.

Top athletes train using high intensity interval training (HIIT), which is a combination of compound exercises that tax both the aerobic and anaerobic systems, while keeping the intensity over 80 percent of your maximum heart rate. It combines short work periods with short rest periods. It's the best way to simulate competition.

HIIT sessions usually don't last longer than 20 to 30 minutes not including your dynamic warm-up and cool down. This may seem like a very short space of time but believe me; if you do the workout correctly, you will be exhausted by the end of it.

There are many different interval variations that you can do (30 second, 60 second, etc.), but one of my favorite types of high intensity interval training is Tabata training. Tabata interval training is the **single most effective type of high intensity interval training**. It is also the **most intense** by far, and surprisingly its the shortest in duration, it **only last for four minutes**... but those four minutes produce remarkable effects. It will probably feel like **the longest four minutes of your life**.

If you are going to try it I would recommend *going light* with the weights, maybe just bodyweight to start, until you find your range. There's a good chance you will underestimate this workout and be begging people around you to help you off the floor.

Tabata intervals follow this structure:

- Push hard for 20 seconds
- Rest for 10 seconds
- Repeat this eight times

The secret to making this effective is in your sprint/work interval. You have to go all out, so **do as many reps as you can in the 20 seconds**, rest for 10, then pick it up again and go all out for another 20 seconds. I recommend choosing 8 different exercises, but there are many ways you can structure this. I would also suggest getting some sort of tabata timer like a watch where you can see exactly where you are in the workout, you don't want to have to think too much, all of your concentration will be on the exercise.

Work your way up to four or five rounds of tabatas with about two to three minutes rest in between each round. This is not a daily workout. If you are capable of doing this every day, you are doing it wrong.

Whatever you decide to do, whether its tabatas or any other variation, high intensity interval training with compound exercises will cut your time in half at the gym by increasing the efficiency of your workout and give you better results in a much shorter period of time.

And the best part about interval training is the fact that it increases energy expenditure during AND after the exercise period, due to a boost in your metabolic rate. This is much better and more effective than your 5 mile jog.

So, to sum everything up, training like an athlete with proper preparation, incorporating total body movements, and increasing the intensity and efficiency of your workouts is a fun way to train, and will break the monotony of your 'routine.' Along with that, you can expect to perform better and look better too – with a body that is as sleek and powerful as you always wanted.

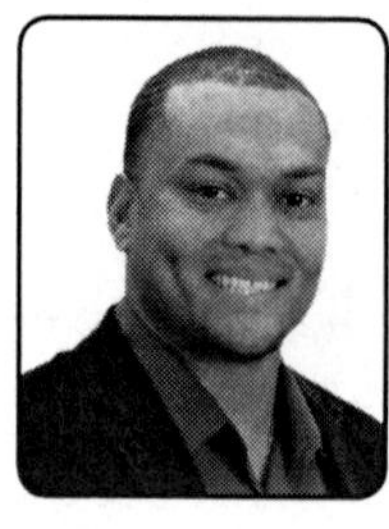

ABOUT VAUGHN:

Vaughn Bethell is a Performance Enhancement Specialist based in Greenville, SC who has worked with many elite-level athletes ranging from high school to the professional ranks as well as over 1000 fitness clients. Many of Vaughn's athletes have gone on to play at numerous colleges and many professional organizations including: NFL, MLS, WPS, A-League, MISL, NBA, etc.

Bethell attended Furman University – where he earned a degree in Health and Exercise Science, as well as being a four year starter with the soccer team, which was ranked in the Division I Top 20 nationally all four years of his career including an Elite Eight appearance and a number 5 national ranking in 1999.

Born in Nassau, Bahamas and raised in Lakeland, FL, Vaughn was also a starter for the Bahamas National Team that took part in the Germany 2006 and South Africa 2010, World Cup Qualifying competitions.

Backed by a formal education and a lifetime of experience and research, Vaughn and his team of former college and professional athletes not only understand the concepts of human performance, but also the science behind it. Vaughn is constantly studying the latest training and nutritional research in order to continually improve his client's physical and mental performance. His goal is to help people find the athlete that lies within them no matter what age they are.

Vaughn is a highly sought after speaker on topics relating to fitness, performance, and nutrition, as well as growth and leadership. To learn more about Vaughn Bethell, visit www.VaughnBethell.com.

CHAPTER 24

TRUTH UNTOLD: FIVE BIGGEST MYTHS ABOUT WOMEN AND WEIGHT TRAINING

BY SHONDELLE SOLOMON-MILES, M.S. (ED) – SPORTS MEDICINE, CSCS

'I don't want to get bulky'/'I don't want to turn my fat into muscle'/'I don't lift heavy weights because I only want to 'tone'. How about this one? …'I only do crunches because I want to flatten my stomach.' If I had a dollar for every time a woman used one of these reasons to justify why she doesn't lift 'challenging' weight, I'd be a very rich woman. Although the growth of female athletics has made strength training more popular among women, and it is not quite as taboo as it was 20 years ago, it amazes me how many misconceptions and outright lies still exist about women who lift weights, especially with all the current research that proves weight training is beneficial for women.

Traditional (and persistent) gender roles, which view strength and muscularity as male characteristics, have a lot to do with the social stigma that women should not lift weights. As a result, many women do not incorporate strength training into their exercise routine, and many who do, approach it incorrectly. Just last week I watched a women at the local YMCA complete a 'weight lifting' workout of at least 100 arm curls and 100 shoulder presses using 3-lb. dumbbells. I'm sure in her mind she was 'toning' her muscles. In my mind, she was wasting time. However, what is more disturbing is knowing that she's not alone. Unfortunately, there are many women 'working out' in gyms right now, who are just as mislead and misinformed. It is my intention then, to highlight the five most common myths women have about weight training, so you will not be one of those women.

MYTH #1
LIFTING HEAVY WEIGHTS WILL MAKE ME BULKY

A woman came into my studio last week for a trial workout. She was 52 years old and seemed to be in pretty decent shape. Her workout consisted of a five-exercise circuit: jump rope, body weight squats, pushups, Russian twists, and barbell shoulder presses. She did not object to any part of the workout - until she had to do shoulder presses with a 25-lb. barbell. While pointing to a ten-pound bar she said: "Can I do this with that bar? This is too much weight and I don't want to get big muscles."

Here we go again.

I've been lifting weights for nearly 12-years, and I have never once been told I look too 'manly'. In fact, when women come into my studio and I ask them how they want to look, they often point their finger at me and respond 'like you.' I don't say this to boast, but to prove a point – women can lift weights and still maintain their femininity.

The fear of a masculine, muscle-bound physique is the most prevalent myth regarding females and weight training. The irony is that the average women should worry more about not having enough muscle, rather than too much. Why? Plain and simple: the more muscle you have, the faster your metabolism and the more fat you are able to burn.

Ladies, please don't be fooled by the women you see on the covers of muscle magazine or even occasionally at your local gym. These women make their living from looking the way that they do, and trust me when I say that building huge muscles does not happen by mistake. It requires a lot of time, calories and steroids for these women to look this way.

There are several reasons why you don't have to worry about 'accidentally' becoming the next 'she-woman'. One, women don't naturally produce enough testosterone, which is the hormone largely responsible for one's ability to "bulk up". In fact, according to several resources, women have about 10 to 20 times less testosterone than men. Therefore, it is very difficult for the average woman to produce 'Arnold Schwarzenegger-sized' muscles by incorporating regular resistance training into their exercise program.

Another reason you don't have to worry about the 'bulk factor' is that gaining size requires a high volume of 'work' for each muscle group. For example, performing 4 sets of 10 squats, 4 sets of 10 leg presses and 4 sets of 10 leg extensions would yield 120 total reps for your quads and hamstrings alone (front and back of thighs). This *volume* of training causes muscle damage and consequently muscle growth. Compare this to a circuit training routine where you combine three or four exercises for three or four different muscle groups. Where. You may include only 3 sets of 8 squats into this circuit for a total of 24 reps. 24 reps versus 140. No wonder bodybuilders spend so many hours in the gym training each day.

One final explanation as to why you don't have to worry about waking up one morning with biceps the size of tree trunks is because building enormous muscles requires eating an enormous amount of calories. Eat more than you burn and you will gain weight, eat less than you burn and you will lose weight. Period. In other words, you can lift weights until the 'cows come home', if you're not eating enough calories to support muscle growth, you have absolutely nothing to worry about.

The Bottom Line: Ladies, lifting weights (and heavy weights) will NOT make you 'big', 'bulky', blocky' or 'buff'. What it WILL do is help you to lose fat, boost your metabolism, shape your body and increase your strength. Who doesn't want that?

MYTH #2
TO 'TONE' YOUR BODY, YOU SHOULD USE LIGHT WEIGHTS AND PERFORM HIGH REPETITIONS.

If you've subscribed to the myth that lifting heavy weights will make you bulky, then you probably also believe that using lighter weights and higher repetitions is the way to 'tone' your body. I call it having a case of the 'Pink Dumbbell' syndrome, and it plagues women in gyms all around the world. I guess this myth appears to 'solve' the problem for all the women who fear that lifting heavy weights will make them 'big'.

First, allow me to clarify the use of the word 'tone'. 'Toning' is a term that has no scientific basis. Muscle tone refers to a muscle's ability to remain contracted under resistance. When you walk up a flight of stairs or lift a box off the floor, you're using muscle tone. Unless you're paralyzed or your muscles have atrophied (decreased in size) to the point of disuse, you already have toned muscles.

What most people mean when they say they want to tone their muscles is that they want more definition and shape to their muscles. In other words, they want less fat covering their muscles so that the muscle is visible. Am I right? Right.

What you truly desire is not toned muscles, but defined muscles - and the only way you'll sculpt or define your muscles is by lifting weight and reducing your body fat. Allow me to briefly explain. Your body composition (how much fat you have as compared to how much muscle) determines how you look. Despite what many people believe, muscle does NOT weigh more than fat, but it does occupy less space, in other words, muscle is denser than fat. This means that if you *replace* (not convert) the fat on your thighs with the same weight in muscle, your thighs will look firmer, slimmer and shapelier.

So is lifting lighter weights and using higher reps more efficient at building muscle and burning fat, than using lower reps and higher loads?

Absolutely Not!

Consider this. If your weight is too light, then your muscles aren't stimulated enough to grow, strengthen, or change in any way. They remain the same (not what you want). If your muscles are already strong enough to do 20 repetitions of a shoulder press with five-pound dumbbells, then your body doesn't need to become any stronger or build any more muscle if you only use five-pound dumbbells.

However, if you begin lifting fifteen-pound dumbbells, your body will have to build more muscle in order to accommodate this heavier weight. As a result, your muscle content will increase, which is one of the desired goals of fat loss, because muscle burns fat. THE MORE MUSCLE YOU HAVE, THE MORE FAT YOUR BODY IS ABLE TO BURN.

In addition, effective fat loss isn't only about how much fat you burn *during* your workout, but how much fat your body continues to burn *after* your workout. This principle is called EPOC (excess post-exercise oxygen consumption), and in very simple terms it refers to the work your body has to do after a strenuous workout to get it back into its 'normal' state. If your weight is too light, EPOC is negligible, and so is your 'post workout' fat-burning potential.

This does not mean that all of your workouts will require you to lift heavy weights, and in fact I encourage you to use a combination of heavy weight/low reps and lighter weight/higher reps (not light). What's most important is that each workout challenges your body beyond its daily demands.

Bottom Line: Changing your body requires a new stimulus; the greater the stimulus the greater the change. If your weights are too light, there is no new stimulus and therefore no change in the muscle. If your muscles do not change you will not improve your body's ability to burn fat.

MYTH #3
WEIGHT LIFTING CAN HELP YOU LOSE WEIGHT IN A SPECIFIC AREA OF YOUR BODY

If you go into any gym across the world, and ask any woman doing crunches why she is doing them, you'll hear some version of: "I want to flatten my stomach." Unfortunately, what these women think they're doing isn't the same as what's really happening.

The belief that you can reduce a specific area of your body by exercising only that area is referred to as spot reduction and it does not exist.

It's critical that you GET what I'm saying here: you cannot choose what area of your body you lose fat from, by exercising that specific area. There is only one exception to this rule and it's called *liposuction*.

I don't care if you do 100, 200 or even 500 crunches a day, if you don't burn the fat covering your abdominal muscles, you'll never 'flatten your stomach'. The reality is the 'abs' you are looking for are already there. The problem is: your fat is hiding it. The solution is: less crunches, a 'clean' diet, and increasing your body's fat-burning potential by lifting challenging weights and doing moderate to high intensity cardiovascular exercise (i.e. interval training).

Bottom Line: You cannot burn fat from a specific area of your body by lifting weights that target that area. The *real* reason why you lift weights is to strengthen your muscles, shape your muscles and perhaps most importantly, to increase your overall muscle content so that you can boost your metabolism, turning your body into a 24-hour fat burning machine.

MYTH #4
STRENGTH TRAINING TURNS FAT INTO MUSCLE.

Think bananas and grapes (I would have said apples and oranges but everyone says that). Just as bananas can't be made into grapes or grapes into bananas, fat can't become muscle and vice versa. **Fat and muscle are two different types of tissue and one cannot and will not ever turn one into the other**. You can gain muscle and you can lose fat, but you cannot ever transform fat into muscle!

If you stop lifting weights, your muscles will atrophy (you'll lose muscle), which means your metabolism will decrease, because your body will not be as efficient at burning calories. Assuming your diet doesn't change to compensate for this slower metabolism, you will gain fat. Again, it's not that your muscle turned to fat, it's that you lost muscle, and as a result, *gained* fat.

Contrary to this scenario, when you begin weight training you are not *converting* your fat into muscle, but rather *replacing* your fat with muscle. In other words, you've lost fat and gained muscle. Remember, muscle takes up less space than fat, so this is why many women report fitting into smaller clothes with consistent weight training, even though they haven't lost any weight on the scale; their body composition has shifted in favor of muscle.

The bottom line – Fat doesn't become muscle and muscle does not turn into fat. Consistent and effective weight training, however, will allow you to lose fat and gain muscle.

MYTH 5
IF WEIGHT LOSS IS MY GOAL, CARDIO EXERCISE IS MORE IMPORTANT THAN LIFTING WEIGHTS.

No, No, No! Eliminating weight training from your fat loss exercise program is a guaranteed recipe for disaster. In fact, along with skipping meals and overindulging in sugar, neglecting weight training is fat loss suicide. I think women have a tendency to gravitate toward 'cardio' activities such as running, biking and elliptical training because it does not pose a threat of getting 'bulky' and cardio machines are easy to use. Not to mention that cardio typically makes you sweat, and many people believe the more you sweat the more weight you lose (another myth by the way, so throw those plastic running suits away).

The problem with the 'cardio-only' mindset however, is that cardio exercise does very little to build muscle, and second, 'cardio' doesn't help you preserve muscle while you attempt to lose fat. When you do *only* 'cardio' exercise and ignore weight training, especially on a reduced calorie diet, you'll lose some fat, but you'll also lose a significant amount of muscle. **Remember, the goal is never to lose muscle. Muscle is your metabolic engine!**

You may think that by weight training before losing weight/fat you'll become thicker and bulkier, but this isn't what happens, because as I previously explained, fat does not turn *into* muscle, muscle *replaces* the fat.

Bottom Line: Fat loss is best accomplished when cardio exercise, weight training and a healthy, supportive diet are incorporated together.

Okay, so there you have it, the five most common myths women have about weight-training debunked. Hopefully, now that you understand that there are more benefits to lifting weights than not, you'll be inspired to grab some dumbbells, train HARD, and become the lean, sexy, fat-burning machine you desire and deserve to be!

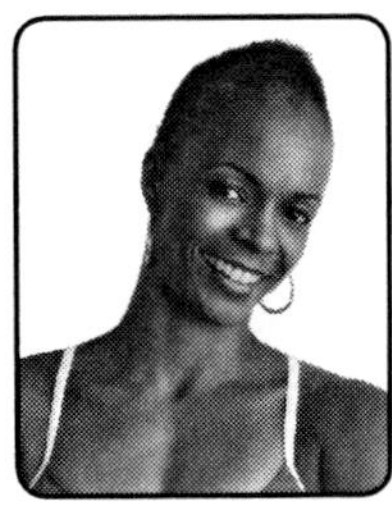

ABOUT SHONDELLE

Shondelle Solomon-Miles discovered her passion for fitness and body transformation upon graduating from Columbia University in 1996, after having worked in the university gym throughout her latter years of college. Since then, it has been Shondelle's personal and professional mission to improve and transform lives via the vehicle of health and fitness. In 2006 years after graduating with her Masters in Sports Medicine from University of Miami, Shondelle established Synergize!, a multifaceted small-group personal training center specializing in body fat loss and weight management for adult men and women. 'I wanted to create an affordable and results-driven alternative to traditional health clubs and one-on-one personal training. I really wanted to help people get lasting, life changing, 'jaw-dropping', results and most of all, have fun doing it." Shondelle says. In June of 2009, Shondelle discovered CrossFit after months of neglecting her own personal fitness regimen, and after experiencing the effectiveness of the CrossFit training methodology, became a CrossFit affiliate in April 2011. 'I've never been more passionate about anything as I am about CrossFit. I love it because it strengthens the mind just as much, if not more so, than the body.'

Synergize! home of CrossFit 954 has since been voted 'Hollywood's best place to workout' for 5 consecutive years by readers of the Hollywood Gazette. Solomon-Miles has also been recognized by the Hollywood Chamber of Commerce as a Small Business Person of the Year Nominee and was voted 'Best 40 Under 40' by *Success South Florida Magazine* in 2008. Shondelle also recently received the honor of 'Fitness Expert of the Year' by the American Business Women's Association.

Author of *The Ultimate Fat Loss Guide*, Solomon-Miles asserts that effective and permanent weight loss is the manifestation of: a healthy mind, a "detoxed" body, supportive nutrition, moderate exercise, effective stress management, and reliable support systems – the six core principles that compose the Synergize! philosophy. Shondelle also believes that misinformation, and lack of enjoyment, intensity and support are the four primary reasons that prevent individuals from attaining their fitness goals, and has made it her mission to help clients overcome these obstacles. Throughout her 15 year career Shondelle has helped well over 3,000 men and women achieve better health and improved physiques by applying her no-nonsense yet fun training methodology. Shondelle resides in Hollywood, Florida with her husband and two young children.

CHAPTER 25

KETTLEBELLS FOR WOMEN'S FAT LOSS

BY ANGELA RAMOS

Five years ago, I woke up and realized I was fat. Perhaps you can relate to this. We, as moms, don't seem to pay much attention to ourselves, our health or our waistlines. Our lives are a whirlwind of activities that leave us little time for exercising or watching what we eat. Meals consist of food left over from our children's plates. Exercise happens when we chase after our kids down the aisles of the grocery store, all the while praying fervently that they won't knock anyone or anything down. Such was the state of my health five years ago. I was a 'stay at home' mom, homeschooling my two older daughters, ages 7 and 13, and chasing after my one year old daughter. I never saw it coming. I did notice that my fourth pregnancy was more taxing on my body than the other three, but I didn't think it had anything to do with my weight.

I became aware of my weight issue when I was watching a video of my first day in the hospital after giving birth to my fourth daughter. I couldn't believe my eyes. I was so overweight and looked swollen. Granted, it was the first day after childbirth but I was still shocked at what I saw. I vowed that I was going to take care of this weight issue as soon as I got the go ahead from my midwife. I knew that I would not keep up with my plan unless I had a partner to hold me accountable. I asked for my husband's help. Due to the type of work he did, there would be weeks where I would need to work out on my own, but if anyone could stay focused, it would be him. So, every morning beginning at 5:00 am, we would work out for an hour and a half, doing a traditional strength training workout 3 days a week and then exercise with a video the other two days, or jog on the treadmill.

With my determination and his accountability, I was able to shed 55 pounds in a year. I was really excited in a new size 6 body and with my newfound energy, but there were still some issues that I had with the traditional weight lifting program I was following. One problem was the hour and a half I was spending every morning working out. It was not a schedule that I would be able to keep up for a long time, especially as my girls got older. The other problem was boredom. I was switching exercises around, but I didn't find my workouts very exciting and they needed some variety.

I'm not exactly sure how I discovered kettlebells, but once I did, they rocked my world. I could get my workouts done in 20 minutes, not an hour doing mindless jogging on the treadmill to get my cardio, and I became even leaner than I was before. I was hooked! I soon became an RKC (Russian Kettlebell Challenge) certified instructor. I now love training other women and helping them get the lean, toned bodies they always wanted.

I'm often asked, what makes kettlebells so special? Can't I get the same benefits by taking an aerobics, pilates or yoga class? I have learned that you cannot use these classes as the base of your fitness program. Okay, seriously, they have their benefits and should definitely be included as supplements to a strength program, but if you want to get lean, strong and toned, you need to think about small cannonballs of iron with handles on them. With that in mind, here are my four reasons you need to start kettlebell training.

REASON ONE:
GET MORE OF YOUR TIME BACK

One of the biggest complaints I get from women is their lack of time. I have to say that it is the main reason I have continued to use kettlebells as the mainstay of my workouts. Kettlebell workouts can be done in as little as 15 minutes and you will burn as many calories or more than the average, traditional strength or cardio workout. That alone makes kettlebell training an awesome tool in a woman's fat loss arsenal. Recently, there was a study done by ACE regarding kettlebell training, where they studied the effects of kettlebell training and the amount of calories burned during a 20 minute workout. What they discovered was that you can burn up to 20.2 calories per minute which is unheard of with any other type of traditional exercise. This allows busy women to get an awesome workout in a short period of time so she can get on with taking care of her family. You eliminate the long workouts and the boring walks on the treadmill.

REASON TWO:
AFFORDABILITY

When my husband and I began working out together, we needed more equipment to do the traditional strength training workouts to which he was accustomed, so we bought a squat rack that had attached cables, Olympic bar, weighted plates, a treadmill, and various sized dumbbells. This was a huge expense of approximately $4,000, and though I still use the equipment every now and then, most of my time is spent with my kettlebells. They are small, take up little room and are much more affordable. In the beginning, you can use just one kettlebell to get your strength and cardio workout done and then add more kettlebells in various weights to keep things progressing.

**Most women should purchase a 12 kilogram kettlebell, which is equivalent to 26 lbs, and the cost is roughly $45. Not bad, huh?

REASON THREE:
INCREASE IN MUSCLE (NOT BULK) = METABOLISM

It always drives me crazy when I meet a new client and I am informed that they never lift anything heavier than five-pound dumbbells because a personal trainer or aerobics instructor told them they would get bulky. Without muscle, you will not increase your metabolism and burn enough body fat to get that lean look you're after. Muscle is not bulky, fat is. It's hard to believe after years of being fed awful lies, but the truth is the more muscle you have, the more calories you burn and the leaner you get. Women need muscle. Muscle is lean and sleek. You want muscle.

Most women's purses weigh at least 20 pounds. I mean, really – think about it! My own mother has a purse the size of 'carryon' luggage. I'm sure her purse weighs at least 50 pounds. Think about how much your children weigh. You are constantly squatting and picking them up every day, so why wouldn't you lift things heavier than five pounds? Women need to get stronger and you do not need to fear muscle. You will not look like Arnold Schwarzenegger, I promise.

Kettlebells allow you to gain strength and add muscle tone while burning off the fat lying on top of your muscles. It's an awesome thing. So, while you exercise for only 20 minutes a day, you can get everything taken care of. Spaghetti arms, jiggly thighs and rubbery abs could be a thing of the past.

Another benefit of lifting something heavy is that you get stronger. Most women who begin training with me have difficulty lifting anything over their heads that's heavier than 10 lbs. and they can't perform a real push-up. One month of kettlebell training improves your strength – enough that you can perform manly push-ups and lift at least 25 lbs over your head. It's true because it happened to me!

REASON FOUR: BRING FUN BACK TO YOUR WORKOUTS

Most women like variety, myself included. Traditional weight training does not offer much variety other than changing from a front lunge to a reverse lunge. A seated military press to a standing military press, etc. After a while, your workouts lack the flair they once did or you plateau. You begin missing a workout here or there. Your intensity and focus begin to waiver. Kettlebells offer so many variations that it is highly unlikely you will ever repeat the same workout twice in a given year. Just for fun, do a search on YouTube for kettlebell exercises and you will see what I mean.

One thing I love to do is combine kettlebell and bodyweight exercises in one workout. I can get a lot of bang for my 20 minutes of work by doing this. Think of bodyweight exercises from your gym classes in school. I like to add jumping jacks, burpees, push-ups, chin-ups, jumping lunges, sprints or squats along with my strength exercises with the kettlebell. Workouts should never be boring and the more unusual they are, the more fun you will have.

Kettlebells are also perfect for exercising outside. I love being outdoors and my neighbors probably think I'm a nut case when they see me throwing or pulling my kettlebells and running around the yard, but I have a great time and the routines are never boring. I recently read a great book by Dan John, *Never Let Go,* where he encourages you to take a look at what you already own in equipment and just create spontaneous workouts utilizing each one once. I've done that and I truly have tons of fun when I do.

It's not uncommon for me to use these spontaneous workouts for my clients at the studio or at my fitness camps, because they were fun to do and quite effective. I make sure the workouts change every time and are fun, while at the same time making sure it helps women shed ugly body fat *fast*. An example of a crazy, thrown-together workout I did was with a 20 kilogram (44 lb) kettlebell, an exercise band and my kid's jungle gym.

- Walk about 20 yards holding the kettlebell at my left side (Farmer's Walk)
- Perform 10 burpees
- Walk the 20 yards back holding the kettlebell on the right side (Farmer's Walk)
- Perform as many chin-ups as I could on the jungle gym, using the exercise band to help me

Kettlebells are an awesome addition to any woman's workout arsenal.

If you want to decrease the amount of time you workout while getting better results, you can't go wrong with the kettlebell. I have never been able to get as lean with a traditional weight-lifting program in only 20 minutes a day as I have with my new preferred piece of equipment. Workouts become fun, spontaneous and effective.

WORKOUTS TO GET YOU STARTED

Here are a couple of quick workouts that take no more than 20 minutes so you can get on with your life:

20 MINUTES OF BLISS (BEGINNER/INTERMEDIATE)

Set a timer for 20 minutes and try to complete as many rounds as you can with as little rest as you can. You cannot rest until you finish all 4 exercises. Try to rest no more than a minute.

Turkish Get Up x 3L/3R
Swing x 20
Clean and Press x 5L/5R
Goblet Squat x 5 (hold for 3 seconds at the bottom)

DOUBLE TROUBLE (BEGINNER/INTERMEDIATE/ADVANCED)

Set a timer for 8 minutes. Complete as many rounds of the circuit until time is up. Rest for 2 minutes before you move on to circuit two.

CIRCUIT ONE (8 MINUTES)

Turkish Get Ups x 5L/5R
Swings x 20
REST 2 MINUTES

CIRCUIT TWO (8 MINUTES)

Goblet Squats x 5
Snatches x 10L/10R

2 MINUTE MADNESS (ADVANCED)

Set a timer for 2 minutes. Try to complete all the exercises in 1 minute or less. Your rest time is the remainder of time left before the timer goes off again. Perform 10 rounds.

10 Jump Squats
5 Push Press Left
5 Push Press Right
5 One Hand Swings Left
5 One Hand Swings Right
20 Two Handed Swings

Note: If it takes you longer than 1 minute to complete the exercises, decrease the level of difficulty by substituting easier exercises.

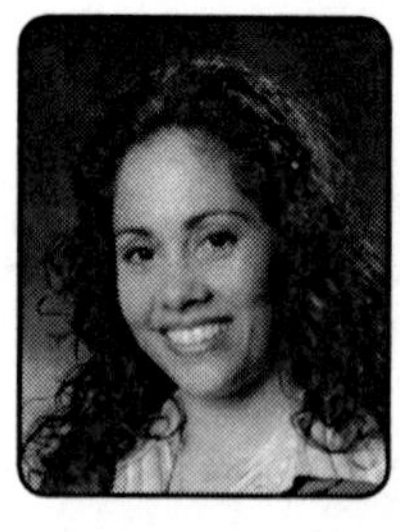

ABOUT ANGELA

For the past five years, Angela Ramos has maintained her initial 55-pound weight loss and has continued to improve her physical health and body composition through kettlebell and fitness training. Since her transformation, she has been committed to helping countless men and women achieve their own body transformation through her scientific fat loss training programs.

Angela received her Certified Fitness Trainer certification from the International Sports Science Association. She is also a Certified Russian Kettlebell Trainer after completing one of the most intense kettlebell certifications with the RKC. She recently was honored to be an Assistant Instructor for the RKC certification in October 2010 in Philadelphia, PA. She is a Certified Back Training Specialist with the CHEK Institute and a Youth Fitness Specialist with the International Youth Conditioning Association.

As a homeschool mom for the last 13 years, she has utilized her experience as a mom with 4 children to create a program just for homeschool moms, The Fit Homeschool Moms Transformation Guide. She reaches the homeschooling masses with a free membership site: www.FitHomeschoolMoms.ning.com.

Angela owns Inspiration Fitness in Crown Point, Indiana, where she and her team of coaches work together to get their clients the best results possible.

"We never settle for 'mediocre' and that is evident in the results, customer service and care our clients receive. We strive to change peoples lives while creating a fun, supportive environment!"

For more information on training, visit Angela's website www.InspirationFitnessCamp.com